NEW ESSENTIAL FIRST-AID

A. WARD GARDNER MD, DIH
and
PETER J. ROYLANCE RD, MB, ChB

A PAN ORIGINAL

Illustrations by
Michael Stokes

Revised and brought up to date

PAN BOOKS LTD · LONDON

First published 1967 by
PAN BOOKS LTD,
33 Tothill Street, London SW1

ISBN 0 330 10646 5

2nd Printing 1968
3rd Printing 1970
4th Printing 1971
5th (Revised and Re-set) Printing 1972

Printed in Great Britain by
Cox & Wyman Ltd, London, Reading and Fakenham

NEW ESSENTIAL FIRST-AID

Dr A. Ward Gardner is a physician specializing in occupational medicine, who works for a major oil company. He has taught first-aid to people with all levels of experience, from doctors and nurses to young school-children, and has produced films and filmstrips on first-aid, safety and accident prevention.

Both as a member of the National Industrial Safety Committee of the Royal Society for the Prevention of Accidents, and in his day-to-day work, he has been involved in safety and accident prevention for many years.

Dr Peter J. Roylance is medical adviser to a leading pharmaceutical group, having previously worked as a research haematologist. In the first-aid and ambulance fields he has lectured to and trained many people and is also active in the Navy reserve.

Both Dr Ward Gardner and Dr Roylance have been actively associated with the work of the Medical Commission on Accident Prevention. They are the authors of *New Advanced First-aid* and *New Safety and First-aid*.

By the same authors in Pan Books:
NEW SAFETY AND FIRST-AID

The Medical Commission on Accident Prevention, 50 Old Brompton Road, London SW7, telephone 01–584–9240, was formed in 1964 by:

The Royal College of Surgeons of England
The Royal College of Physicians of London
The Royal College of Surgeons of Edinburgh
The Royal College of Physicians of Edinburgh
The Royal College of Physicians and Surgeons of Glasgow
The Royal College of Obstetricians and Gynaecologists
The British Medical Association
The Royal College of General Practitioners.

Its aims are 'to establish a medical advisory body to provide information on medical aspects of accident prevention, first-aid and life-saving, and to communicate and publicize the views, findings and reports of the Commission to the public, to Government departments, voluntary societies and other bodies. The Medical Commission on Accident Prevention aims to promote the wider teaching of first-aid and life-saving techniques, and training methods designed to prevent the occurrence of accidents and injuries arising therefrom. The Commission also aims to examine the need for, and to sponsor research in, medical aspects of accident prevention, first-aid and life-saving, and in the physiological and psychological aspects of accident-producing behaviour.'

Contents

Preface

TO THOSE of you who are learning first-aid for the first time, we hope that this book will be of great help.

To those of you who are experts in first-aid, we know that you will find this book different and up to date.

We should like to keep it up to date and would value any suggestion for improving the content, presentation or clarity of the text, or any ideas for improved methods of first-aid or home treatment.

Your comments, observations and criticisms are more than welcome.

If you like this book, or if you don't like it, or if you have any views or ideas and would like to tell us, please write to us at:

Pan Books Limited,
33 Tothill Street,
London, SW1

Acknowledgements

WE WISH to thank all the people who have helped in preparing this book, and are especially grateful to: Dr J. L. J. de Bary; Miss R. Bechtold; Mrs M. L. Birch; Mr Jason G. Brice, FRCS; Ian W. Cameron, FDSRCS; Squadron Leader L. W. Davies; Dr Eric Jones-Evans; Dr Roy Goulding; Mr George Kirkham; Mr J. Ellsworth Laing, FRCS, Ed; Mr L. G. Lewis; Dr J. W. Lloyd; Chief Fire Officer G. Nash, GRAD I FIRE E; Dr J. D. Ogilvie; Dr L. G. C. E. Pugh; Mr P. A. M. Weston, FRCS; Dr Joan Whelan, and Mrs Eve Williams.

We are grateful to everyone who has written to make suggestions for improving this book. In each case we have given careful consideration to the ideas and have adopted a number in this revised edition.

Introduction

THIS BOOK HAS been written to provide an up-to-date view of first-aid. Our aims have been to present first-aid as a subject based on easily understood principles, from which there follows by inference the correct action and treatment. We have also tried to make the subject as simple as possible.

In the excellent book *Principles for First-Aid for the Injured*, Proctor and London (who are surgeons at the Birmingham Accident Hospital) call attention to two principles which should be used in teaching first-aid, and which we have tried to follow in this book:

(1) 'To inculcate a clear appreciation of the order of priority of treatment; to teach dogmatically the most urgent conditions, how they are to be recognized (which may mean looking specially for them) and how they should be treated. Less serious conditions may also require treatment, but in some circumstances they may have to be passed over for the sake of avoiding delay that might prove fatal.'

(2) 'Frills must be eliminated.'
 For example, seriously injured casualties:

  (i) should only have *essential* first-aid which *benefits* them;
  (ii) should not have their arrival in hospital delayed by 'treating' trivialities;
  (iii) should be given NOTHING by mouth EXCEPT if they are seriously burned and conscious (when they should, if adult, be given half a cup of water every ten minutes);
  (iv) should not be heated and are best left cold. When under cover inside a building or an ambulance, cover with one blanket. Never use hot water bottles;
  (v) should be transported swiftly and comfortably to hospital.

There are already a number of books on first-aid – so, why another?

In the course of teaching first-aid, and of reviewing the results of current teaching, we have become aware:

— that many problems are tackled by first-aiders without understanding the principle involved (as distinct from the detail);

— that an excess of instruction can serve to cloud an issue which
is simple in principle;

— that a few simple rules which are remembered and carried out
will tend to be more effective first-aid than half-remembered
floundering;

— that attention to breathing and to airway maintenance is less
well understood and practised than it needs to be;

— that often the best first-aid will be to do a few simple things
effectively and get the casualty comfortably and without delay
to hospital; and

— that the principle of the calculated risk should be accepted.

The principle of the calculated risk is that if the correct and beneficial treatment for a certain condition is, in 99 cases out of 100
(or some such number), to do a certain thing, but that to do this
in 1 case in 100 may result in less favourable or unfortunate
results, we accept the 1:100 risk and act.

The simple rules for the treatment of unconsciousness provide
a good example. These rules are designed to direct attention to
breathing and the airway. The instructions are that all unconscious persons should, after having the mouth cleared quickly of
dentures, loose teeth, blood, vomit or debris, be turned into the
unconscious (semi-prone) position, if possible with a slight head-
down tip. There is no doubt that the great majority of unconscious casualties will benefit by this treatment – indeed there is
evidence that just over 20 per cent of one sample of 200 road
deaths were due to nothing else but blood or vomit blocking the
airway. These, and many other lives could be saved by the application of the simple rules for the treatment of unconsciousness.
There will be an occasional unconscious casualty, however, who
may suffer serious injury by being turned – for example, the
casualty with the broken neck.

The dilemma is whether to teach all the possible exceptions,
with the result that the first-aider becomes confused or spends a
lot of time doing useless checking – which he may or may not do
well or be able to do effectively – instead of getting on with vital
first-aid measures, OR whether to take a calculated risk and teach
a few simple steps which can be easily remembered, and which

should be well carried out, and which in the overwhelming majority of cases will prove to be effective in saving lives. Following the excellent example set by Dr Robert A. Mustard (to whom we are greatly indebted for some ideas in simplifying the approach to first-aid) in the Canadian St John Ambulance first-aid book, *The Fundamentals of First-Aid*, we have throughout this book used the principle of the calculated risk.

We have also assumed that any first-aid will be carried out in a place from where skilled medical help is but a few hours away.

This book is not intended to give instruction in what to do if medical help is unobtainable – for example in lonely parts of the world or at sea. For such circumstances quite a different sort of book is required such as *The Ship Captain's Medical Guide*, *The Ship's Medicine Chest and First-Aid at Sea*, *Exploration Medicine*, or *A Traveller's Guide to Health* (*see* Appendix 3, page 181).

To those who seek such help we recommend these books.

Doctors and first-aid instructors who are used to a more orthodox approach to first-aid may notice the absence of material which traditionally clutters the text of first-aid books. For example, a chapter on the structure and functions of the body. Much of the detailed anatomy and physiology which is given is quite unnecessary for an understanding of first-aid. In order to carry out efficient artificial respiration by the exhaled air method, a few simple instructions are, in our estimation, worth more than any amount of elaborate anatomy and physiology of the respiratory system. Similarly, the 'causes of asphyxia' is a discussion of interest to doctors, but the first-aid problem is:

firstly to recognize whether the casualty is

    1. breathing or not breathing;
    2. conscious or unconscious and breathing.

secondly to apply the simple rules for dealing with a casualty who is

    1. not breathing;
    2. breathing but unconscious.

All elaborate discussion of structure and function, or of differential diagnosis of the causes of not breathing or of unconsciousness, merely detract from a clear understanding by the first-aider of the problems which face him. The first-aider should be led to see the problem in simple terms of 'not breathing' and 'unconsciousness'.

The doctor has quite a different problem: he has to resolve *why* the casualty is not breathing and *why* the casualty is unconscious in order to apply the different forms of treatment for each. But to expect first-aiders to do this – or to burden them with the substance of it – is to trail clouds of confusion. There is plenty of scope for first-aid; but first-aid should be presented to first-aiders in terms of how they will see or recognize the problem and not in medical jargon and differential diagnosis.

We have also omitted all reference to shock and the treatment of shock from our text, for the same reasons as Dr Robert Mustard omitted them from *The Fundamentals of First-Aid*, that 'there is no single important measure which will not be carried out for reasons much more obvious than the treatment of shock'. We would refer our readers to the introduction of Dr Mustard's book if they would like to read a fuller discussion of the reasons for omitting shock and the treatment of shock from first-aid book texts.

Other deliberate omissions include tourniquet; pressure point; Holger Nielson, Schafer and Silvester methods of artificial respiration.

Our hope is that by simplifying instructions what is left will be *essential* and of *benefit* to the casualty and will be *remembered and understood* by the first-aider. The text is, as the title suggests, essential and not advanced first-aid.

Heart compression (closed-chest cardiac massage) has been omitted from this book. We think that it is a technique which is too difficult and potentially dangerous for the occasional or basically trained first-aider. A description of heart compression appears in *New Advanced First-Aid* (*see* Appendix 3, page 181).

Readers who have studied first-aid for many years will find that some procedures which they have been trained to do are no longer required. Good first-aid, which will benefit the casualty, consists of getting priorities right, applying the essential treatment and getting the casualty to hospital without delay. Experienced first-aiders may feel some disappointment at having to do less treatment. However, we hope that the casualty will benefit from this approach, and that experienced first-aiders will remember the educationalist's aphorism 'knowledge is the greatest bar to learning' and will try to see what is useful in this new approach to essential first-aid.

Chapter 1

GENERAL INTRODUCTION
to first-aid and home treatment

Definition of first-aid

First-aid is the process of carrying out the *essential* emergency treatment of an injury or illness in order to *benefit* the casualty. The casualty is then sent to hospital or to a doctor for further treatment. The treatment of the casualty is *not* completed at the scene of the injury. Treatment is initiated with the understanding that further treatment will be required.

Self-help and first-help

FIRST-AID can be divided into two parts:

1. self-help;
2. first-help.

Self-help is what the casualty can do for himself.
First-help is what other people (first-aiders) can do for the casualty.

Home treatment is only-help and not first-aid

Home treatment, which is used for minor injuries and non-serious conditions, could be described as 'only-help'. This is *not* a part of first-aid as we have defined it.

In *first-aid* (which is *self-help* plus *first-help*) the treatment given is initial treatment. The casualty is passed on for further treatment.

The *home treatment* of minor injuries and conditions is full treatment (*only-help*). The casualty is *not* passed on for further treatment. This book is therefore divided into two parts:

I. first-aid (self-help and first-help);
II. a chapter on home treatment (only-help).

		aim of treatment	*to see a doctor for further treatment or observation*
First-aid	1. Self-help	To do all possible for oneself as the casualty	Yes
	2. First-help	To treat the casualty and pass the casualty to someone else for further treatment	Yes
Home treatment	3. Only-help	To carry out full and effective treatment of the injury or condition without sending the casualty to a doctor	No, unless in a few days' time all is not well

SELF-HELP

The traditional idea of first-aid involves an active first-aider and a passive casualty. In many instances, the first form of assistance could and perhaps should come from the casualty himself. Self-help should therefore be taught as a part of first-aid training. Much can usefully be accomplished in stopping bleeding (by direct pressure and by limb elevation), supporting injured parts, summoning help, and moving around by the injured person himself. Indeed in certain circumstances the injured person may have to rely on self-help for some time before first-help arrives. As part of first-aid, the self-help which the injured person can and should give himself may make all the difference.

For example, a person may sustain a broken leg when alone

at home. Two problems will follow – what to do about the broken leg, and how to get help. The injured person could lie on the floor and use pillows, cushions or folded rugs or clothes to support the broken leg. He may have a telephone, and can thus summon help easily – or he may have to yell for help.

A broken arm could be kept against the trunk and supported by the other arm (the good-arm sling, *see* page 109).

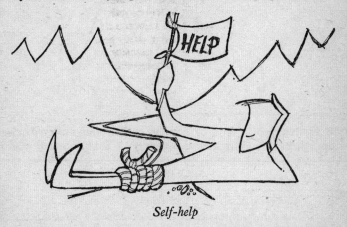

Self-help

In bleeding, the injured person could apply pressure with his fingers to where the blood is coming from and thus stop the bleeding by digital pressure. Such action could even be life-saving in certain circumstances.

In cases where a feeling of faintness comes on, the person could apply self-help by lying down in the unconscious (semi-prone) position and by removing any false teeth.

Another good example of the use of self-help is to allow a casualty with an injured ankle to place himself on a stretcher. The first-aider supports the ankle during the move, and *then* ties the feet and legs together. If this tying is carried out first, the subsequent problem of transfer on to the stretcher is needlessly difficult, especially if the casualty is heavy.

Wounds can be covered, help can often be summoned, and much else can be done by the injured person. These ideas about self-help are an important part of first-aid. We shall include remarks about self-help in every chapter where self-help is, or could be, useful.

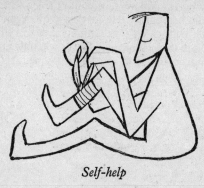

Self-help

Injured people tend to become excited and flustered, or apprehensive and frightened, so apply:

SELF-HELP

> *If you are a casualty, try to remain calm and collected. Think out what you can do to help yourself by self-treatment. Try also to summon assistance from other people.*

The *AIMS* of *FIRST-AID* are to

PRESERVE LIFE. Every other need is secondary to this

MINIMIZE the EFFECTS of INJURY

RELIEVE PAIN and DISTRESS

DELIVER a LIVE CASUALTY in good condition to HOSPITAL

Essential emergency treatment means doing what *must* be done to preserve life and *leaving undone* those things which ought not to be done, in order to get the casualty quickly to hospital in the best possible condition – that is, to benefit the casualty.

First-aid has been defined above as the process of carrying out the *essential* emergency treatment of an injury or illness in order to benefit the casualty before sending the casualty to hospital. Essential emergency treatment must benefit the casualty – for example it would be foolish to delay a waiting ambulance in which was a casualty suffering from serious blood loss (a life-threatening condition) in order to bandage a minor graze on the back of the hand (not a life-threatening condition).

Skilled neglect of unimportant injuries when faced with serious conditions and life-threatening injuries can save lives. Well-judged restraint or masterly inactivity may be the correct treatment in some cases. What *can* or *could* be done and what is *essential* and *must* be done are often quite different. Lack of delay in getting a casualty to hospital may make the difference between life and death.

Provided that the hospitals get a live casualty to treat, there is much that can be done by modern treatment to save lives. A casualty arriving dead cannot be helped by any treatment. The job in first-aid is to deliver a living person to hospital in the best possible condition for further treatment.

In this book, you will find the aims of first-aid for particular conditions such as burns, fractures or unconsciousness, discussed chapter by chapter. An aim which is always present is to 'treat other injuries'. To avoid needless repetition, and to help the clarity of presentation, the aim 'treat other injuries' has not been stated in every chapter. This aim should, however, always be understood to apply.

Chapter 2

PRIORITIES AND THE SYSTEMATIC APPROACH

Priorities

By priorities we mean carrying out the
CORRECT ACTIONS in the
CORRECT ORDER. These actions must be to carry out the
essential treatment which will
benefit the casualty, and then get the casualty quickly to
hospital.

What we *could* do and what we *should* do will, in many cases, be quite different. Correct decisions about priorities are among the most difficult decisions which face any first-aider. However, in any particular incident the order of priorities is usually apparent.

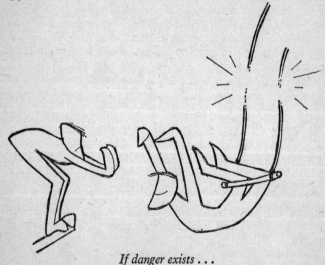

If danger exists . . .

Do what has to be done in the correct order. Then, get the casualty to hospital without delay. Do not delay by 'treating' trivialities.

A SYNOPSIS OF PRIORITIES

1. If danger exists, do not become the next casualty yourself.
2. Remove the casualty if necessary from a position of immediate danger.
3. Check that the casualty is *breathing*.

IF THE CASUALTY IS NOT BREATHING

  (i) Quickly check for and remove any obstruction (dentures, debris, loose natural teeth, blood or vomit), then tilt the head *fully* back.

  (ii) If breathing does not begin at once, start *artificial respiration* (*see* page 41).

4. Stop any severe *bleeding* (*see* page 55).

5. If the casualty is breathing but *unconscious*, turn him into the unconscious (semi-prone) position, check for any possible

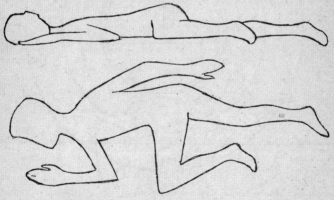

The unconscious position

cause of obstructed breathing (dentures, debris, loose natural teeth, blood or vomit) and apply a slight head-down tip if possible.

The order of doing 2, 3, 4 and 5 will be determined by the

nature of the incident, but the correct order should be obvious in any particular case.

6. Cover all *serious wounds and burns*.

7. Immobilize *broken or dislocated limbs* or *suspected fractures*.

8. *Do not delay* by treating minor injuries or trivialities if serious injuries are present – get the casualty *to hospital* quickly. There are always doctors in hospital.

9. At some stage in above, send for help, giving a clear message. If there are many casualties, sending for help should have a very high priority.

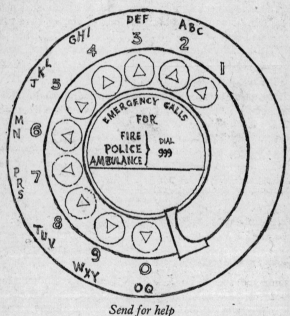

Send for help

THE CALCULATED RISK IN RESCUE

Any would-be rescuer must always weigh up carefully the probable results of any action which he or she may take, *before* taking that action. Bravery implies a calculated risk: foolhardiness is occasionally mistaken for bravery. The situation is made worse if the would-be rescuer becomes the next casualty. For example a party of sailors were returning to their ship late at night and slightly drunk. One of their number, who was known to be a non-swimmer, fell into a dock. Another sailor immediately dived into the dock to rescue his non-swimming colleague. Unfortunately for all concerned, it was a dry dock.

Another example is the casualty in a gas-filled area. If there is enough gas present to overcome one person, anyone else, such as a would-be rescuer, who goes into and remains in the area may be similarly overcome by gas. Therefore, the rescuer must accomplish what he has to do in one breath, taken away from the danger area, or he must wait until someone comes with breathing apparatus who can spend time safely in the gaseous area. Otherwise, the rescuer may be the next casualty.

The caution which is being sounded here may seem to some to be advocating a rather anti-heroic attitude. This is indeed what we are trying to do. The principle of look (and think and calculate) before you leap is a wise one. The work of subsequent rescuers can be made much more difficult by a multiplication of the number of casualties by foolish would-be rescuers. We know of many such cases – and perusal of the newspapers will no doubt continue to bring to light many more similar occasions. Having sounded this note of caution, let us hasten to add that we have also known many fine acts of calculated bravery where a risk was assessed and successful action was taken. So, remember when you reach the danger area to stop, to think and to calculate for a moment; it may make an enormous difference to the outcome.

Sending for help

At some appropriate stage, send for help – from other people, from doctors, for an ambulance, and so on. Try to give a very clear message to the ambulance authorities or the police or the doctor, to include:

  how many casualties;
  what sort of injuries;
  what help you think is needed;
  exactly where you are;
  the telephone number to call you back on.

CORRECT PRIORITIES

A good example of the importance of getting priorities right was a casualty who was found lying on the edge of the road face downwards on top of his moped bicycle. He was blue in the face and *not breathing*, and appeared to be dead. Full neck extension – produced by grasping his hair and pulling the head back as far as it would go – coupled with holding the lower jaw up with the other hand in the teeth-clenched position, produced an immediate inward gasp of air. He had been suffering from *obstructed breathing* (*see* page 38). Artificial respiration was not required. The casualty could not breathe because he had become unconscious and the air passage to the lungs was blocked by the head-forward position. His tongue was blocking the air passage.

At this point a breathless man rushed up and said 'I found him lying there and I've sent for the ambulance.' This man was *not* a first-aider; his priorities were wrong. Sending for the ambulance at this time was not essential and did not benefit the casualty. It would in fact have produced a dead casualty, because the ambulance did not arrive until ten minutes later.

The casualty was now *unconscious but breathing*. The mouth was quickly searched for dentures or loose natural teeth (none found) and the next move was to place the casualty in the unconscious (semi-prone) position (following the rules for the treatment of unconsciousness).

An attempt was then made to turn the casualty into the unconscious position, but it was discovered that his right index finger was caught between the chain and the rear-drive sprocket of the cycle. How then to get the casualty into the unconscious position? The answer was to turn the pedals of the bicycle and thus free the end of the index finger. As both hands were being used to keep the head back and the lower jaw supported, the breathless newly-arrived man was asked to turn the pedals. His face showed clearly what he thought – 'what, and mince the casualty's finger-end?' In a voice of stern authority he was instructed to turn the pedals – and did so! A finger-end is of less importance than the life-saving correct treatment for unconsciousness. (Little damage was in fact done to the finger-end.)

The casualty was now placed in the unconscious position and within four minutes had recovered sufficiently to talk. He was allowed to sit up just before the ambulance arrived some five minutes later. A head injury was found during a rapid examination while he lay recovering in the unconscious position. It was this head injury which started the chain of events leading to unconsciousness and obstructed breathing, from which he very nearly lost his life.

There are many lessons to learn from this story. We hope that by reading it you will remember the importance of correct *priorities* and of doing the *essential* things to *benefit* the casualty – that is, the *correct actions* in the *correct order*.

Removal to hospital and the questions of speed and comfort
Many casualties are rushed to hospital and suffer unnecessary discomfort and aggravation of their injuries as a result of a fast ride. Others, suffering from serious life-threatening injuries have their arrival in hospital delayed by excessive attention to trivial injuries prior to loading into the ambulance. How is it possible to find the correct balance between speed and comfort to use as a practical guide?

Unfortunately it is not easy to make simple rules. Each case must be decided on its merits. However, in the table on the next page, the medical condition of the casualty is given together with the relative importance of speed and comfort.

THE BY-MOUTH RULE IN FIRST-AID
Give NOTHING *by mouth except to conscious burned casualties or to some conscious poisoned casualties.*

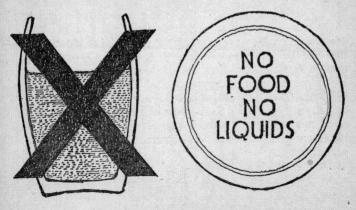

NO
FOOD
NO
LIQUIDS

Injuries or Condition	Comments	Action
Serious multiple injuries.	May easily die, and probably needs blood replacement.	NO DELAY TOLERABLE. IGNORE MINOR INJURIES. GET CASUALTY TO HOSPITAL SOON.
Head injury, getting more deeply unconscious.	May easily die.	
Serious bleeding.	Needs blood replacement.	
Unconscious, following poisoning.	Only hospital treatment can help.	
Fractured thigh.	Could need blood transfusion.	PROCEED WITH REASONABLE SPEED. TREAT MINOR INJURIES, BUT DO NOT DELAY UNDULY. ATTEND TO THE COMFORT OF THE CASUALTY.
Fracture of both ankles.	Comfort important—not life-threatening.	
Fracture of both wrists.	Comfort more important than speed.	
Dislocated shoulder.	Comfort more important than speed.	
Head injury, showing signs of recovery.	If any signs of deterioration, then there must be no delay.	
Fractured pelvis.	Comfort important; sometimes life-threatening from severe internal bleeding.	
Fracture of the spine.	Do not hurry. Careless handling could lead to very serious consequences. Must go slowly and carefully.	MUST NOT HURRY. COMFORT IMPORTANT.

The reasons for this rule are:

(i) All *unconscious casualties* and all casualties with *chest and abdominal injuries* should be given NOTHING by mouth because it may choke or further injure them.

(ii) Many casualties will require an *anaesthetic* shortly after arrival in hospital – and for this it is best to have an empty stomach – so NOTHING should be given by mouth.

(iii) *Burned casualties* will lose fluid from their body by leaking through the areas of burned skin (by weeping, or by forming blisters). This fluid loss can be a very serious problem and corrective steps should be taken at the earliest possible moment – as a first-aid measure – to deal with the problem. *Conscious* burned casualties should be given half a cup of water every ten minutes (*see* page 93 for details). *Unconscious*

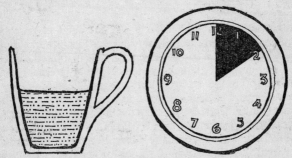

Give conscious *burned casualties half a cup of water every ten minutes*

burned casualties, like any other unconscious casualty, should be given NOTHING by mouth.

(iv) *Conscious poisoned casualties*. After the casualty has been made to vomit, he should, if adult, be given 2–3 glasses of water (or other bland fluid) to dilute any remaining poison (*see* page 147 for details).

THE ONE-BLANKET RULE IN FIRST-AID

One blanket is all that is required to conserve body heat in a casualty who is inside a building, in an ambulance, or in a sheltered place.

The aim of using a blanket is to prevent heat loss and

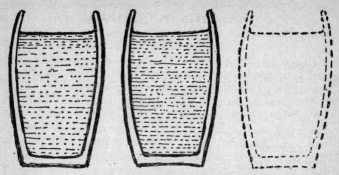

Some conscious *poisoned casualties after being made to vomit are given 2–3 glasses of water (or milk, lemonade, etc)*

conserve normal body heat; it is not intended to raise body temperature. Overheating – by whatever means – of seriously injured casualties is bad treatment. Seriously injured casualties are often in need of blood, due to external or internal bleeding (including around fractures). Following blood loss, the remaining blood is channelled round the vital parts of the body (brain, lungs, heart) by shutting down circulation through the skin. For this reason, the skin is pale and cold, and the casualty will feel cold and may actually shiver. Because this sensation of shiveryness and coldness is a self-protective mechanism it should *not* be interfered with by heating the casualty. The casualty should be left to shiver and feel cold.

Hot water bottles and overheated rooms should be avoided. Of course on cold floors and such surfaces a blanket should also be used under the casualty. Out of doors, there may be a need for more covering, but the number of blankets should be kept to a minimum.

THE SYSTEMATIC APPROACH

In first-aid, as in many other things, there is a need to have a systematic approach to problems. On page 29 there is a scheme which sets out the main points to be covered systematically in first-help.

THE SYSTEMATIC APPROACH

Approach ↓	Calm, reassuring, announce that you are a first-aider.
Appraisal of the situation ↓	Danger? How many casualties? Help required? How to summon help? How long before help arrives? Time to get casualties to hospital? What help is available?

Quick appraisal
of casualty
↓
	Priorities?
	  Breathing?
	  Bleeding?
	  Unconscious?

Life-saving first-aid if required ↓	
Detailed appraisal of casualty ↓	History – talk to casualty, ask what he feels is wrong with him. Examination – looking and feeling.
Diagnosis ↓	What is the matter?
First-aid to prevent worsening ↓	Essential and to benefit the casualty.
Removal	To hospital.

1. *Approach*

A calm and reassuring and relatively unhurried manner will do much to allay anxiety or fear – and most injured people are afraid. Perhaps the best way to see this need clearly is to picture the extreme opposite, when a casualty finds a hot, flustered, excitable person bearing down on him. Such an approach does not inspire trust, confidence or a belief in the competence of the so-called first-aider! Always try to calm yourself before approaching a casualty or an incident.

It is also important to announce that you are a trained first-aider. This reassures the injured person and other helpers who may be present. There are occasions when doctors or nurses may also be present to give first-aid.

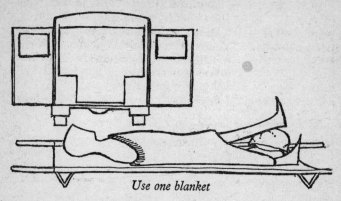

Use one blanket

2. *Appraisal of the situation*

Answers to questions such as 'is there further danger?' or 'what time will the journey to hospital take?' may make a difference as to how the situation is handled. A fuller discussion of these points appears at the end of the book in Chapter 12, page 155.

3. *Quick appraisal of casualty*

Having decided to treat one casualty, the course to follow will depend on the priorities, that is on whether the casualty is:

   (i) Breathing or not breathing.
  (ii) Bleeding or not bleeding.
 (iii) Conscious or unconscious,
        and so on.

4. *Detailed appraisal of casualty*

   (a) *History* – the casualty's story of what happened

In the case of conscious casualties, you should begin by asking them what they feel is the matter (the complaint) and go on to find out what happened and how the injury occurred. This process of questioning a casualty to find out what he feels to be wrong with him and how the injury was sustained is known as taking the history – and the substance of the story is the history of the injury or illness.

In certain circumstances, for example if a casualty is unconscious, confused or cannot remember what happened, a useful history of the injury or illness can often be obtained from witnesses of the incident and from bystanders. Always ask and accept all the help you can get in this way – the clues may enable you to suspect or to guess intelligently what is the matter with the casualty. A careful history will often reveal more useful information than an examination of the casualty.

(b) Examination – looking and feeling

In first-aid, looking and feeling are the main ways of examining a casualty to find out what is right or wrong. Never forget that most people are symmetrical about the mid-line and that they have two arms and two legs! Always use the good side to compare with the bad. If you do not know what is the normal shape, say of a casualty's ankle, look at the uninjured one and compare the good with the injured one.

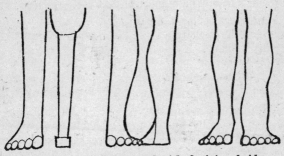

Always compare the good with the injured side

When feeling for tenderness or examining for pain (for example, moving a joint) always look at the casualty's *face* and not at the part which you are examining. You will usually learn much more about pain and tenderness in this way than by asking questions – the answer should be apparent from the casualty's face.

5. *Diagnosis* – what is the matter?

Diagnosis is a medical word which means 'this is what the casualty is suffering from'. To make a diagnosis, all the previous information should be carefully collected and thought about. Then, it should be possible to decide what is the matter – the diagnosis. Without correct diagnosis, treatment becomes akin to shooting in the dark. If we know what is the matter, we then know what to do. If we do not know what is the matter, or have only a vague idea, or *fail to find out* by lack of careful history-taking or examination, we are unlikely to give the best form of treatment. A thorough and methodical attempt to find out what is the matter will usually give sufficient information to guide treatment, even in the absence of an exact diagnosis.

6. *Removal*

In first-aid, the casualty will always be passed on to a doctor for further management because first-aid means first (aid) treatment. There are a number of choices:

   (i) Bring the doctor to the casualty.
  (ii) Send the casualty
     (*a*) walking
     (*b*) by car
     (*c*) by ambulance

    to hospital or to a doctor.

In cases which are urgent, serious or doubtful, the best removal is generally by the first available transport or by ambulance, to the nearest hospital for accident cases. There are always doctors in hospital, and in hospital all the extra help in terms of people and equipment is available for the casualty.

Giving information

Giving information to the casualty or to relatives may often be a problem. In general, it is better initially to say too little than too much, and wiser to give hope than to give over-optimistic prophecies. It is also much better to admit ignorance than to give bad or misleading information. Wild and uninformed

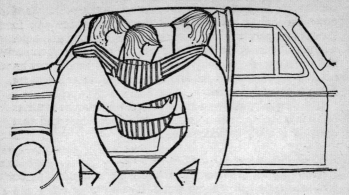

Send the casualty to hospital by the first available suitable transport

guesses merely create further distress for the casualty and for his relatives, and more problems for doctors.

A note on gentle handling

The importance of the gentle and careful handling of any casualty, particularly of a severely injured casualty, cannot be overstressed. Rough handling increases pain and apprehension, and can make injuries considerably worse or bleeding more severe. In good first-aid, there is no place for panic handling. For example, we have seen a casualty being scooped up and dumped on to a stretcher, then bumped into the ambulance and driven off with little attempt to find out what is the matter, to apply first-aid or to be gentle. This sort of panic handling of casualties only makes matters worse and increases the severity of any injuries. Gentleness is important in all aspects of first-aid, for example, in examining the casualty to find out what is the matter or in applying splints and slings to fractured limbs.

Treating the person as well as treating the injuries or illness

Injured or ill people are often frightened and in pain. They require comfort and reassurance in addition to treatment of their injuries or illness. The good first-aider will convey his concern for the casualty's well-being by speaking kindly and quietly to him as he carries out the necessary first-aid. In serious incidents involving many casualties the good first-aider will not discuss grisly details but will try to give reassurance and convey to the casualty that he is in good hands, that his needs as a person are seen, and that his injuries or illness are being adequately treated.

If the casualty asks you about others, who may be relatives or friends, tell him that you are doing your best and that everyone is being helped.

Extrication of a casualty from wreckage

Injured people, whether in wreckage or not, need to be handled gently and without panic. If you cannot easily and gently remove a casualty from, for example, a smashed car, you should leave him where he is and do your best to treat him there until help arrives *unless* there is imminent danger.

Forceful extrication should be carried out only if further danger threatens. There is no point in making existing injuries needlessly worse by the use of force in removing a casualty if he would come to no immediate harm by being left.

Always mention trapped casualties when calling for help. Fire brigades are usually able to deal with the extrication of trapped casualties. Remember to ask for all the help which may be needed – from ambulance, police, fire brigade or others – when making the *first* request for help.

Chapter 3

NOT BREATHING

Preamble

Correctly applied first-aid can be immediately life-saving in three conditions:

NOT BREATHING
BLEEDING
UNCONSCIOUSNESS

This chapter is devoted to a discussion of the problem of not breathing, and the next two chapters deal with first-aid for bleeding and for unconsciousness respectively. We have headed these chapters 'life-saving first-aid' because of the potential for saving lives which exists when the correct first-aid is carried out for not breathing, for bleeding and for unconsciousness. However, lives can also be saved by 'first-aid to prevent worsening', a heading which should be applied to the remaining chapters about first-aid.

How to recognize that a person is not breathing

Listen with your ear close to the casualty's nose and mouth for breathing. Even if there is a lot of noise you will be able to *feel* his breath in your ear.

Look for movement of the chest or of the upper part of the abdomen, where the ribs divide at the lower end of the breastbone.

Breathing may stop as a result of

head injuries
unconsciousness from any cause
electrocution
gassing
poisoning
drowning
  or other reason.

However, these reasons can all be seen to act through one or both of two basic reasons.

The basic reasons for not breathing are:

(i) *Obstructed breathing*

In this condition, the air passages between the lungs and the outside are blocked, and because of this obstruction, the casualty cannot shift air in and out of the lungs – that is, he cannot breathe.

(ii) *Brain malfunctioning*

For normal breathing movements to occur, the brain must send out regular signals to the muscles which produce breathing movements. If, through head injury, lack of oxygen, poisoning or other reason the parts of the brain which control breathing do not send out regular or correct signals, air will not be shifted in and out of the lungs at all, or may be shifted in inadequate amounts.

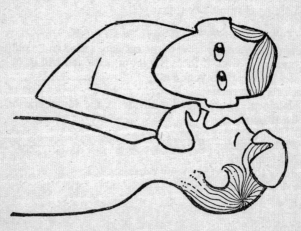

Listen for breathing

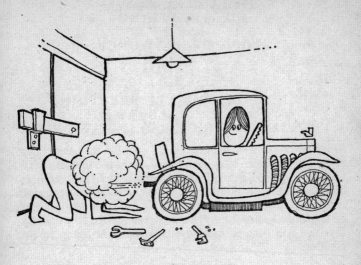

A common cause of gassing – the garage doors are shut

Reason for not breathing	*Remedy in first-aid*
obstructed breathing	relieve obstructed breathing
brain malfunctioning	give artificial respiration by mouth-to-nose or mouth-to-mouth method

The *AIMS* of *FIRST-AID* for *NOT BREATHING* are to

Relieve obstructed breathing and, if the casualty does not breathe at once, to
Give artificial respiration.

Giving artificial respiration means shifting air in and out of the lungs of a person who cannot breathe naturally, by doing the work of normal breathing for him.

The fact that any casualty is
NOT BREATHING
must be
RECOGNIZED AT ONCE.
There must be
NO DELAY
in applying first-aid to
RELIEVE OBSTRUCTED BREATHING
and if breathing does not begin at once in
GIVING ARTIFICIAL RESPIRATION

When anyone stops breathing, his life will be in the balance, for about four to six minutes at the most, from the time at which breathing stops. Because these emergencies often occur suddenly, and because you will have to act quickly to be successful, *it is essential that you know exactly what to do and that you have often practised doing it before the emergency arises.* It is unlikely that you will succeed unless you do the right things in the right order.

Obstructed breathing

The two main conditions which result in obstructed breathing are

Unconsciousness
Fluids or solids blocking the air passages

The conditions may occur together or separately.

1. *Unconsciousness*

Any person who becomes unconscious *for any reason* may be unable to move. If the unconscious person is lying on his back – and particularly if his head is pushed forward by a pillow – the jaw and tongue may sag backwards and *the tongue can thus block the air passage at the back of the throat* (*see* top figure on page 39).
   This may be the only reason why an unconscious person cannot breathe.

2. *Fluids or solids blocking the air passages*

Blood, vomit or saliva can easily form a fluid seal and block the back of the throat – especially if the tongue has fallen back,

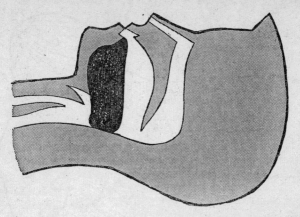

In an unconscious casualty the tongue may block the throat

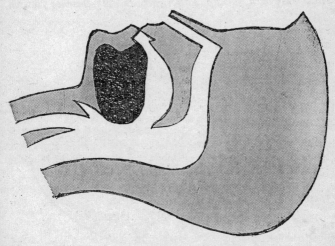

Normal clear airway in a conscious person

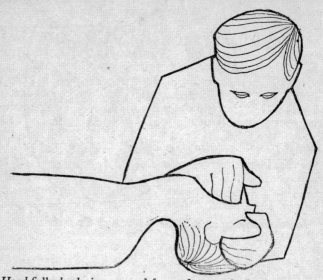

Head fully back, jaw up and forwards to teeth-clenched position

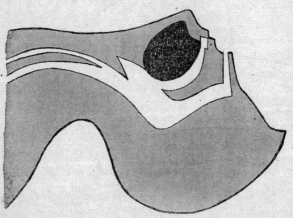

In this position the air passages are clear and unobstructed

narrowing but not quite blocking the air passage. Dentures, debris or half-swallowed objects may also block the air passages.

Unconscious people may also be unable to swallow, cough or spit and thus are unable to clear the blockage. The combination of unconsciousness with lying on the back and either bleeding from the mouth and nose or vomiting is particularly liable to produce obstructed breathing and is potentially fatal. A conscious person will not suffer in this way but an unconscious person can easily die from obstructed breathing.

How to relieve obstructed breathing

The condition is simply remedied – *pull the head back firmly as far as it will go,* and at the same time, *bring the lower jaw upwards and forwards* to the upper jaw until the front teeth meet. This can be called the teeth-clenched position. In this position, with an undamaged jaw, the tongue cannot fall back and block the air passages. Make sure that you bend the head back fully. Bend the head backwards until it will go no farther. It is surprising to many people how far back the head will go with *full* neck extension.

It may also be necessary to *clear the mouth and throat* quickly of anything else which may cause obstruction of the air passages such as false teeth, loose natural teeth, blood, vomit or debris. Use a clean handkerchief or a paper tissue to blot out blood and vomit from the mouth and throat. If you have nothing else, use your finger to scoop out blood clot and vomit. If the casualty does not breathe immediately after bending the head back and clearing the mouth and throat, then you must proceed at once to the next step, which is to give artificial respiration.

Artificial respiration

The aim of artificial respiration is to do the work of normal breathing for a person who cannot breathe naturally, thus shifting air in and out of his lungs.

Artificial respiration should be given by breathing air directly into the casualty's lungs through the nose or mouth.

Exhaled air is quite adequate to ensure that sufficient

oxygen reaches the casualty. Fresh air contains about $\frac{4}{5}$ nitrogen, $\frac{1}{5}$ oxygen, and just a trace of carbon dioxide. Exhaled air contains the same amount of nitrogen, a little more carbon dioxide and a little less oxygen, but there is still sufficient oxygen for effective artificial respiration.

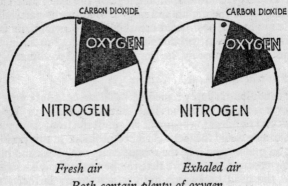

Fresh air   *Exhaled air*
Both contain plenty of oxygen

Air can be breathed into the lungs by blowing through the casualty's nose, through the casualty's mouth, or in the case of infants and small children, by blowing through both the nose and the mouth at the same time.

In adults, the mouth-to-nose method is best, because there is less danger of inflating the stomach and causing regurgitation of stomach contents, thus producing vomiting. In poisoned casualties it is safer to use mouth-to-nose breathing as the rescuer will be less likely to come in contact with poison from the lips of the casualty.

How to do artificial respiration

In order to carry out artificial respiration it is necessary to:
1. Act immediately.
2. Have a clear and unblocked air passage from the nose or mouth to the lungs.
3. Shift air in and out of the lungs.
4. Continue to apply artificial respiration until the casualty breathes.
5. Turn the casualty, when he is breathing regularly, into

the unconscious (semi-prone) position. He will still be unconscious when he starts to breathe and all unconscious casualties must be placed in the unconscious position, with a slight head-down tip if possible.

6. Watch carefully to see that the casualty continues to breathe.

7. Arrange for the casualty to be taken to hospital, still watching carefully to see that breathing is maintained.

8. If the casualty stops breathing again, start artificial respiration at once.

1. *Act immediately.*

Unless breathing of good air is continuous, the vital centres in the brain are soon damaged by lack of oxygen. Within four to six minutes from the time of cessation of breathing the casualty will be beyond recovery unless air passes in and out of the lungs. Speed is vital: life depends upon it. Start artificial respiration at the earliest possible moment. There is, for example, no point in taking a drowned person quickly to dry land if in the intervening period he could be given artificial respiration in a boat, or if a few lung inflations could be given in waist-deep water. Every second counts: begin artificial respiration at the earliest possible moment.

2. *Have a clear and unblocked air passage from the nose or mouth to the lungs.*

Obstructed breathing must be remedied (*see* page 41) before air can be blown into the casualty's lungs.

3. *Shift air in and out of the lungs.*

This is done by breathing (blowing) deeply and slowly through the casualty's nose, while at the same time blocking off the mouth, until the casualty's chest is seen to rise. Having delivered a good inflation, the rescuer then removes his mouth from the casualty's nose and allows the air to escape from the casualty's lungs. The rescuer should turn his head to watch the chest falling and to avoid the casualty's exhaled air. When all the air has escaped, the rescuer should again blow to inflate the casualty's lungs and allow the air to escape. Make absolutely sure that the chest rises each time you breathe into the

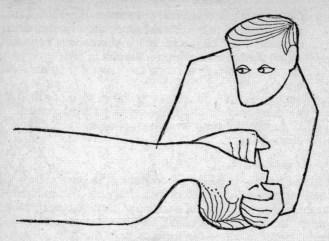

Head fully back

1. If possible have casualty on back. Tilt head firmly backwards as far as it will go. Rapidly remove dentures, debris, blood, vomit or loose natural teeth.

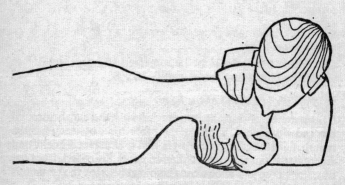

Inflate

2. Breathe deeply and slowly into casualty's nose, keeping his lips closed with your thumb. If nose is blocked, breathe through his mouth keeping his nostrils pinched. The chest will rise as it fills with air.

casualty. Be sure also that you have an airtight seal between your mouth and the casualty's nose or mouth so that air does not escape when you blow. Continue in this manner until the casualty breathes by himself, or for at least an hour.

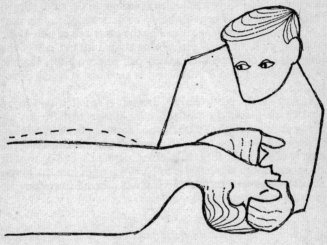

Watch chest falling

3. Take your mouth away and relax. The chest will fall. Inflate again. If the chest does not rise and fall, check head and neck position as in Fig 1. Continue for at least an hour.

If for any reason mouth-to-nose artificial respiration cannot be carried out – for example because the casualty's nose is blocked – then use mouth-to-mouth. One or other of these two methods can always be used, and will succeed in shifting air into the lungs. The first choice is mouth-to-nose, but no time should be lost in changing to blowing through the mouth if mouth-to-nose breathing does not inflate the lungs.

In infants and very young children, after securing full neck extension, the rescuer should cover with his mouth *both* the nose and mouth of the infant. Gentle puffs only should be used – just sufficient to secure a good rise of the chest.

If the heart is beating, the first inflations should produce an improvement in the colour of the casualty – from blueness, or blue-greyness, towards pinkness. The first six to ten inflations should be given as rapidly as possible.

The rhythm of subsequent inflations should be allowed to determine itself. Give a full inflation, allow all the air to escape, then begin again. The rate should be determined in this way, by the casualty's own needs *and* by the casualty's colour. If the colour is pink, sufficient air is being shifted in and out of the lungs. If the colour is blue or very pale or grey, either the rate or depth of inflation is insufficient or the heart is failing or not beating.

In some cases, particularly in drowning, or following gassing by irritant gases, the casualty may appear to have his air passages full of froth. You cannot remove this froth by wiping, so do not waste time trying to remove it. As this froth consists largely of *air* in the form of bubbles, all you have to do to shift air in and out of the lungs is to blow the froth into the lungs. So, blow as usual. In this way you will succeed in shifting air into the casualty's lungs.

4. *Continue to apply artificial respiration until the casualty breathes*

When the casualty starts to breathe by himself, the breaths will be shallow and weak. The rescuer should time his inflations to coincide with the casualty's own weak breaths, and should continue to assist the breathing until it is judged that breathing is satisfactory.

The rescuer should apply artificial respiration to a casualty who is not breathing for not less than an hour or until told to stop by a doctor.

5. *Turn the casualty when breathing into the unconscious position*

When the casualty is breathing, the situation will be that of an unconscious but breathing casualty. Following the rules for unconsciousness, the casualty should, therefore, be turned into the unconscious position and, if possible, be placed with a slight head-down tip (*see* Chapter 5, page 71).

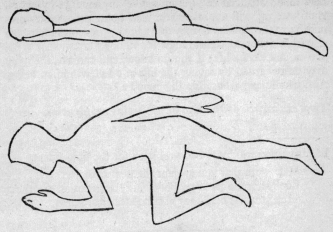

The unconscious position

6. *Watch carefully to see that the casualty continues to breathe*

Once a casualty has started to breathe there is no guarantee that he will continue to do so. Watch carefully for any signs of weakening of breathing. If you judge that breathing is weak, turn the casualty on to his back and recommence artificial respiration to assist natural breathing. If breathing stops, turn the casualty on to his back and commence artificial respiration again.

7. *Arrange for the casualty to be taken to hospital*

Do not be in too much of a hurry to move the casualty. Although the casualty needs to be in hospital as quickly as possible, make sure that natural breathing is well established before attempting to move him. This will ensure a live casualty arriving at the hospital. Continue to watch carefully during the journey and be prepared to start artificial respiration again at any time. Transport should, of course, be in the unconscious position with a slight head-down tip.

A note about practice

Be sure to practise how to relieve obstructed breathing and

how to do artificial respiration *before* any emergency arises. Half-knowing will not save lives. Half-doing these procedures may harm the casualty or may lose a life by preventing someone else from doing the right things. If you don't know what to do, you cannot save a life; if you do know, and can act, then you may be rewarded by saving the life of a fellow human being. And who knows whose life this may be?

Two examples of the use of artificial respiration

Electrocution

Electrocution produces two problems for the first-aider:

1. Make sure that you are not the next casualty.
2. Look after the casualty. Following electrocution breathing often stops. There may also be electrical burns.

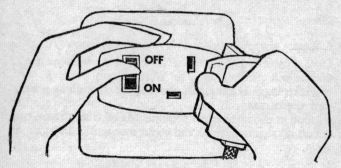

Switch off and remove the plug

Make sure that you can approach safely

Before approaching any electrocuted casualty, make sure that it is safe for you to do so – check that the current is off or that the casualty is now out of contact with the source of current, and that you will not be endangered by your approach. If you cannot switch the current off, ease the casualty from the electricity supply with an insulated lever. Remember that water is a good conductor of electricity and use only dry material. Do not touch the casualty's moist armpits.

When approach is safe, check breathing

Having made certain that you can safely approach the casualty, check to see that the casualty is breathing. If not breathing, commence artificial respiration at once. Continue artificial respiration until the casualty breathes on his own.

When or if breathing, place the casualty in the unconscious position:

The casualty will then be unconscious but breathing, so turn him into the unconscious position and apply a slight head-down tip if possible.

Then, treat any burns and send to hospital:

Quickly cover any burned areas (*see* Chapter 7, page 92). Remove the casualty to hospital, checking the breathing continuously during the journey.

Always seek help:

At some time early in the above list of priorities, help should be sent for or sought.

Drowning

Make no attempt to drain fluid out of the lungs. Such attempts are useless.
Start artificial respiration at the earliest possible moment – in shallow water, in a boat, or at the water's edge.
Continue for at least an hour.
When breathing commences, use gentle puffs to aid weak breathing.
Turn the casualty into the unconscious position with a slight head-down tip if possible.
Send to hospital as soon as normal breathing is established. Watch carefully all the way to hospital and be ready to start artificial respiration again at any time.

Footnote

Many people have been trained in artificial respiration using the exhaled-air (mouth-to-nose or mouth-to-mouth) method. The step which seems to be most easily forgotten or most poorly carried out is concerned with having a clear and

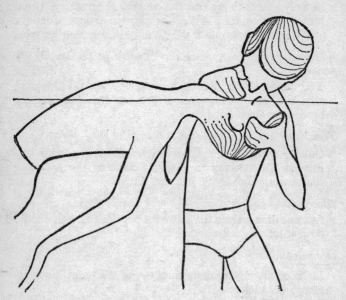

Start artificial respiration at the earliest possible moment

unobstructed air passage from the nose or mouth to the lungs –
see again how to relieve obstructed breathing (page 41). Make
sure, by re-reading, and by looking again at the illustrations on
pages 39 and 40, that you do not forget the need to have a *clear
unobstructed air passage* and *the head fully back before you start
to blow*.

Some people may find that the close contact with an often
unknown and apparently dead person is unpleasant. This can
be overcome by blowing through a pocket handkerchief which
is used to cover the casualty's nose and mouth.

Summary of first-aid for NOT BREATHING

Life-Saving First-Aid I

Check for breathing ⟶ · *Listen* with ear over nose and mouth
Look at lower chest and upper abdomen for movement ⟶ **BREATHING**

NOT BREATHING
↓
Relieve OBSTRUCTED BREATHING — Remove blood, vomit, dentures and debris, bend head back as far as it will go and support lower jaw in teeth-clenched position ⟶ **BREATHING**

NOT BREATHING
↓
Give artificial respiration ⟶ Use mouth-to-nose or mouth-to-mouth methods. Continue for one hour at least ⟶ **BREATHING**

NOT BREATHING
↓
After one hour, probably dead. Continue to give artificial respiration until you to stop or until you are sure the casualty is dead

Place the casualty in the UNCONSCIOUS POSITION with a slight head-down tip, CHECK for and TREAT any SERIOUS INJURIES and SEND to HOSPITAL. Watch carefully in case breathing stops again

Chapter 4

BLEEDING AND WOUNDS

BLEEDING

Bleeding means loss of blood *from the circulation*. Blood which cannot be circulated is not useful to the body. Only blood which circulates can carry out the proper functions of blood, such as carrying oxygen around the body. If blood is lost from the circulation in other than small quantities, this blood must be replaced SOON.

Bleeding may be:

1. *External* – when blood escapes from the circulation *to the outside of* the body.
2. *Internal* – when blood escapes from the circulation *inside* the body.

    Internal bleeding may be:
    (i) *Visible*, when the blood can be seen, for example, by being coughed up or vomited.
    (ii) *Concealed*, when the blood cannot be seen.

1. *External bleeding*

This can usually be seen and recognized. However it may be necessary to search for bleeding, particularly underneath the body in places like the hollow of the back, behind the knee and in the buttock area.

2. *Internal bleeding*

Examples of bleeding inside the body are:

(a) Bleeding which occurs around the ends of broken bones. Considerable amounts of blood may be lost to the circulation in this way. The swelling which appears around the site of broken bones is due to bleeding.

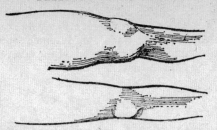

The swelling around a fracture is due to bleeding

(b) Bleeding into body cavities such as the chest or abdomen.

(i) *Visible internal bleeding* is blood which arises from inside the body and is brought to the outside of the body, for example by coughing from the lungs, by vomiting from the stomach, by trickling from the ear or nose when the skull is fractured, or by passing blood in the urine or motions. A bruise is also an example of visible internal bleeding.

(ii) *Concealed internal bleeding* is equally serious, but is more difficult to diagnose. Bleeding can take place, for example, from the brain, liver, stomach, spleen or around fractures. Three or four pints of blood can quickly be lost without being seen.

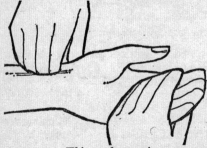

Write down the pulse rate and the time at five-minute intervals in all cases of suspected internal bleeding. A pulse rate which rises as time passes is an indication that bleeding is continuing.

This needs practice

How to recognize concealed internal bleeding
You must be able to recognize that the casualty is bleeding, even though you cannot see any blood. He will look ill and *pale*, although this may be difficult to see in dark-skinned

people. The skin will be colder than normal, especially the hands and feet. Often the skin feels clammy due to sweating. The pulse will usually be rapid – for example, over 90 beats per minute – and feeble. It can be felt at the outer side of the wrist by the tips of the fingers.

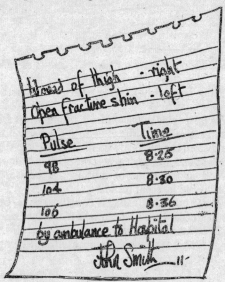

A useful note to hospital from a first-aider

No time must be wasted in getting casualties who are bleeding or who have bled to hospital. Blood loss needs blood replacement in hospital – SOON.

The amount of blood loss

Adults can lose one pint of blood from the circulation slowly without suffering any severe effects, as is well known by all blood donors who give to the blood bank.

However, there is a limit to the amount of blood which can be lost without causing trouble. It is perhaps stating the obvious, but nonetheless worth saying, that *the greater the amount of blood loss, the greater is the threat to the casualty's life or immediate well-being*. And again, that blood loss, if serious, needs blood replacement – SOON. Blood loss in external bleeding can be estimated from the amount of blood which is spilled or from bloodstaining on the clothes. Any loss of over 2 pints in an *adult* begins to be serious. *Much smaller amounts are dangerous in children.* In internal bleeding which occurs around broken bones, the size of the swelling will give a clue to the amount of blood loss. A broken thigh in an adult will usually result in a loss from the circulation of *at least* 2 pints and a broken shin bone *at least* 1 pint. If these two injuries are present together, the total blood lost to the circulation will be *at least* 3 pints. If, in addition, there are other injuries such as wounds which have bled externally (say ½ pint), and a broken elbow (say ½ pint), the casualty may be first seen when he has already lost 4–6 pints of blood from the circulation. Such casualties need blood replacement – SOON. The amount of blood loss from concealed internal bleeding can only be estimated by the general appearance and from the pulse rate.

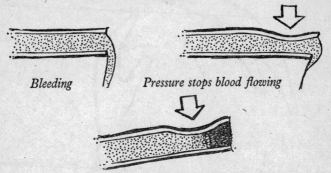

Bleeding   *Pressure stops blood flowing*

Pressure plus rest and elevation help to form a clot

The AIMS of FIRST-AID for BLEEDING are to:

Stop bleeding quickly.

Bleeding ceases naturally when blood stops *flowing* and forms a *clot*. First-aid should therefore aim to stop blood flowing (by pressure and by elevation) and should aid clot formation by rest, because movement breaks up the clot.

Send the casualty to hospital without delay, in case blood replacement is required.

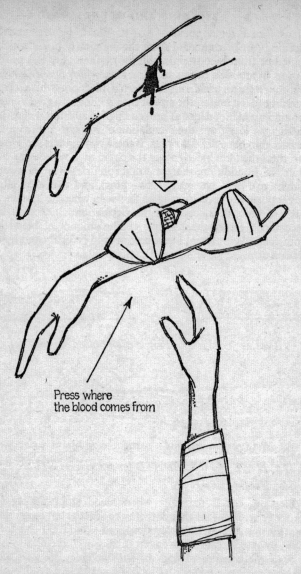

Press where
the blood comes from

How to stop bleeding from a cut on the forearm.

How to stop external bleeding

1. Apply firm pressure directly over the bleeding area or wound. Use a sterile dressing if possible. If not, use anything clean. Use your hand and fingers if nothing else is available. Pressure with the fingers on or around the wound can always be used to stop bleeding. In emergency, do not waste time looking for dressings: put your finger or your hand on the bleeding spot and press. This should stop the bleeding until you can apply a dressing.

2. If the wound continues to bleed through a dressing apply *another* pad and bandage over the first and tie slightly tighter or apply more pressure by hand over the wound. *Do not* remove existing dressings as this will only disturb blood clot which has formed and make bleeding worse.

3. If bleeding is from a limb, elevate the limb unless it is broken and you would do more harm by moving the limb.

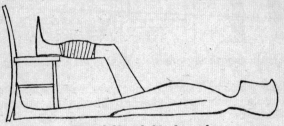

Wound dressed, leg elevated

4. Rest the injured part so that blood clot which is formed will not be disturbed, thus giving rise to renewed bleeding.

5. Reassure the casualty and tell him to lie quietly. Agitated casualties do not lie still and therefore tend to bleed more. This advice should be given in ALL cases of bleeding or suspected bleeding.

6. Casualties who have bled more than a small amount should have the lower limbs elevated, if other injuries permit. This transfers blood from the legs to the heart and brain, where the blood is most needed.

7. Send the casualty to hospital, watching carefully that bleeding does not start again. Watch especially the general condition, the pulse rate and any wounds from which the casualty

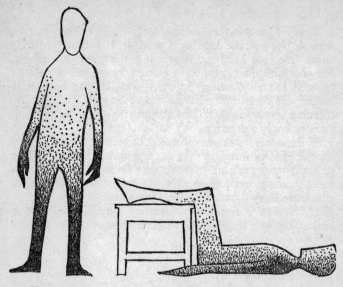

Elevation of the legs transfers blood to the heart and brain

could lose blood without this being noticed easily – for example by bleeding underneath clothes or by bleeding from the under-surface of the body.

How to treat internal bleeding

There is no first-aid measure which can stop internal bleeding. The first-aid treatment of internal bleeding has therefore to be directed firstly towards helping nature to stop the bleeding by *rest*, and secondly towards getting the casualty to *hospital* where special treatment can be given to stop the bleeding and to replace blood loss.

Any casualty who is thought to be suffering from internal bleeding should therefore be put at rest, usually lying down, and should be sent swiftly to hospital.

Chest injuries with internal bleeding should be transported to hospital in a sitting or half sitting-up position (*see* pages 129 and 130).

Self-help in bleeding

This can be a valuable – even life-saving – procedure. The illustrations on page 60 show how self-help could be carried out.

Always try to remain calm in an emergency, and try to get your priorities right. In bleeding, the first priority will be to stop the bleeding. Next, summon help. If you feel that you may faint or become unconscious, lie down in the unconscious position and try to lie in such a way that you can continue pressure on the bleeding area – for example by lying on the injured side or by pressing your fist into the wound and lying on that arm and elbow in such a way that your own weight will keep the pressure up even if you do faint.

WOUNDS

A wound is any break in the skin or other body surface which arises from injury. A skin graze or a cut inside the cheek are examples of a wound.

The AIMS of FIRST-AID for WOUNDS are to:

Stop bleeding (keep blood in).
Prevent infection (keep germs out).

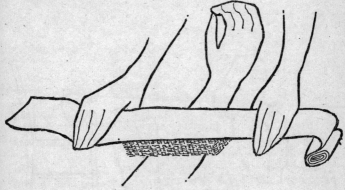

Apply a sterile dressing

(i) *Stop bleeding*

How to stop bleeding is dealt with above. The instructions can

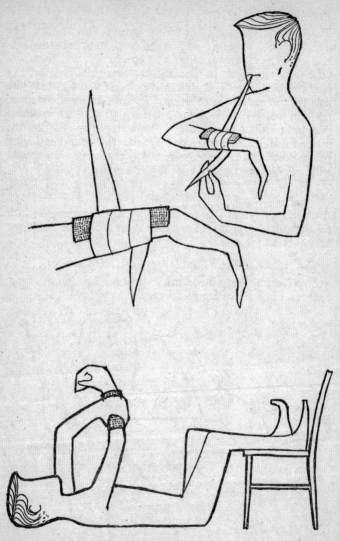

Self-help in bleeding

be summarized as follows: for external bleeding, press where the blood comes from and elevate limbs; for internal bleeding, send the casualty to hospital.

(ii) *Prevent infection*

Everything which comes into contact with the wound should if possible be sterile. If possible do not touch the wound even with washed hands. Use sterile dressings. Put the sterile dressings on to the wound without touching the surface of the dressing which will be next to the wound with your hand. Try not to cough on, or breathe over, wounds or sterile dressings. Once dressings are in place do not take them off again. When wounds have been dressed to stop bleeding and to prevent infection the first-aid treatment is over except to transport the casualty to hospital quickly.

Foreign Bodies

A foreign body is any material or substance which should not be in a wound or inside the body, for example, dirt, grit, sand, wood, glass or metal (which may be found in wounds or in the eye) and coins, beads or safety pins (which may be swallowed by children or lodged in the ear passage or nose). Foreign bodies may be large or small, single or multiple.

In first-aid the rules about foreign bodies are:

Remove loose foreign bodies and leave alone any foreign
bodies which do not lift easily out of the wound.
Never attempt to prise or force foreign bodies out of wounds.

If there is:

   (i) a foreign body which does not lift easily out of the
      wound, or
  (ii) a fracture at the site of bleeding (especially a fracture of
      the skull when bone fragments may be pressed into and
      damage the brain),

build up dressings in and around the wound and then apply pressure to the edge of the wound. In this way you will stop the bleeding without causing further damage.

Some examples of first-aid for bleeding

1. *Bleeding from a wound*

(i) *Lay the casualty down.*

The casualty may faint from sudden loss of blood, so tell the casualty to lie down before he could faint.

(ii) *Press with your hand or finger* on the bleeding spot if bleeding is severe.

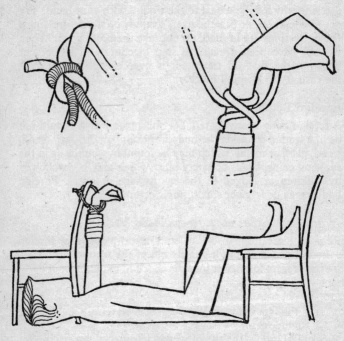

Elevate the limb

(iii) *Elevate if bleeding is from a limb.*

Unless a limb is broken, the limb should be raised. This helps to stop the bleeding until pressure can be applied to the wound. Raise the lower limbs where permissible in all casualties who have lost blood. This transfers blood from the legs to the heart and brain.

(iv) *Remove clothing*.

Damp clothing stained dark red usually means bleeding. Remove sufficient clothing to see all the wound. This enables you to see the full extent of the damage and to estimate how much bleeding is taking place. Large superficial wounds usually bleed far less than small deep penetrating wounds.

Remember to examine the rest of the casualty for bleeding. Severe bleeding is not always painful or obvious. Look or feel under the casualty for any dampness. Until you can show clearly that any dampness is *not* due to blood, you must assume that it is due to bleeding. Casualties are still found who have bled to death quietly from wounds under themselves which were not sought and recognized.

(v) *Look at the wound, remove any loose foreign bodies or lumps of dirt*.

Look for glass, metal, wood and other foreign bodies. If the foreign body is loose remove it without touching the wound. Road gravel, soil or other fine dirt in the wound is best left alone in first-aid.

(vi) *Cover the wound*.

Dressings must be built up around any foreign bodies or broken bone ends so that when the bandage is applied, pressure is applied all round the wound but not on the foreign body or broken bone ends. If no fragments of foreign material or broken bone ends are in the wounds, a sterile dressing can be applied directly on to and completely covering the wound. Sterile dressings are usually pre-packed and must be opened carefully without touching, breathing or coughing on to the dressing (*see* page 81). If sterile dressings are not available, an unused, freshly washed and ironed handkerchief or other items of clean linen make a good substitute. Put plenty of gauze or padding over the dressing. This makes sure that pressure is comfortably applied to the wound when a firm bandage is applied. A sterile dressing pressed on to the wound may hurt but it will stop bleeding.

A crêpe bandage is easily the best bandage to apply. It will hold the dressing in position and apply useful pressure. A cotton bandage is not so good as it does not apply pressure as evenly or as well as a crêpe bandage. If the bleeding is from an arm wound, after applying the dressing (pad and bandage) apply a triangular (St John) sling (page 84). This rests the injured part, thus preventing further bleeding which may arise due to clot breakdown by movement. It also increases comfort.

Dressings which are used to stop bleeding from wounds should be checked at intervals to ensure that there is no further bleeding. *Under no circumstances should dressings be removed and re-applied on the way to hospital.* Lives have been lost following the removal and replacement of a dressing. Because a wound has stopped bleeding when a dressing is taken down *is not* a guarantee that the bleeding will not start again. Bleeding which soaks through a dressing should be controlled by further dress-

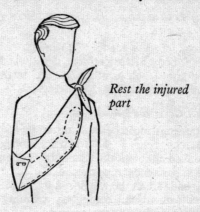

Rest the injured part

ings, more pressure and limb elevation. Watch closely the general condition of any casualty who is thought to be bleeding. The pulse rate and time should be recorded at frequent intervals. A rise in the pulse rate with time is a sign of continuing bleeding. Bleeding should be sought for especially on the underside of wounds and dressings, and underneath the casualty. Any dampness should be thought of as possible bleeding until proved otherwise.

(vii) Reassure the casualty that bleeding has stopped.

Injured people are frightened people until they are told that they will be all right. Restless casualties disturb blood clotting and thus bleed more.

(viii) Send the casualty to hospital as soon as possible. Even though you have stopped severe bleeding, blood loss needs to be replaced swiftly by blood transfusion, and hospital is the place for this.

2. *Bleeding from the nose*

This is often caused by over-enthusiastic blowing or by an injury to the nose. Self-help and first-help are the same. Sit the casualty down with his head well forward over a basin or bowl. Tell him to pinch all the soft lower part of the nose firmly for

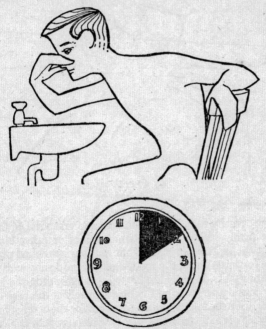

Pinch the lower soft part of the nose for 10 minutes by the clock

10 minutes timed by the clock. Release slowly – if any blood flows, repeat the pressure again for another 5 minutes before releasing again. If bleeding still continues send the casualty to hospital in a sitting position, holding his nose.

3. *Bleeding from the lip or cheek*

This is often caused by the teeth. Sit the casualty down and tell him to clench the damaged region with a gauze dressing held firmly between thumb and finger. Here is one region where pressure can be applied on *both* sides. Self-help is usually best – but this procedure can also be used by the first-aider.

Then send the casualty to hospital.

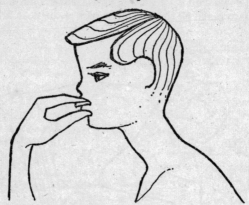

Press on both sides

4. *Bleeding from the tongue*

Tell the casualty to put out his tongue and grasp the end of the tongue firmly, using a clean handkerchief or other cloth to prevent the fingers slipping off the wet surface. Now pull the tongue forwards out of the mouth gently and firmly as far as it can comfortably be pulled. This will probably stop the bleeding by causing pressure on the blood vessels at the base of the tongue. Keep the tongue pulled forwards for about ten minutes. Release slowly and check that bleeding has stopped. If bleeding continues, pull the tongue forwards again.

In addition, a pad may be pressed over any wound that can be reached. Press on *both* sides of the wound.

Self-help to stop bleeding from the tongue can be given by the casualty himself pulling the tongue as far out as it will go. This will usually stop the bleeding.

5. *Bleeding from a tooth socket*

This kind of bleeding is seldom serious. At least two-thirds of the 'blood' spat out will be saliva – so there should be no need for panic about the amount of blood loss.

Fold or roll a clean handkerchief or similar clean piece of cloth and fit the end of this across the tooth socket between the adjacent teeth. Allow any excess of material to hang out of the corner of the mouth. Tell the casualty to bite firmly onto the cloth. The firmness of the bite may cause discomfort but should not be so tight as to cause pain. Keep biting for 20 minutes, timed by the clock. Release the pressure slowly. Remove the cloth carefully and gently so as not to disturb clot formation.

If bleeding continues, repeat pressure with a cloth and continue biting – but for a little longer this time. Should this fail to stop the bleeding, re-apply pressure and seek further help. Remember, however, that the amount of blood loss is usually slight and that there should not be any need for alarm or panic.

6. *Bleeding from the ear passage*

This kind of bleeding is usually caused by blast or by head injury. Lay the casualty down. Place a loose pad over the affected ear and bandage it in place – not too firmly. Keep the affected ear *downwards*. If he is unconscious treat as any unconscious casualty by placing him in the unconscious position with a slight head-down tip AND with the bleeding ear *downwards*.

7. *Bleeding from an amputation*

Lay the casualty down. Elevate the remaining part. Apply a dressing to the stump and bandage tightly in order to exert *very* firm pressure on the stump. If bleeding continues, build up further dressings and apply firm pressure with the hand over the end of the stump. This is one situation where *really firm pressure* may be required *both around and over* the end of the stump in order to stop bleeding.

8. *Black eye*

A black eye is a bruise of the eye socket and lids. The colour and swelling are due to visible internal bleeding. In the early stages, ice packs can help to prevent swelling. When the lids are closed by swelling (blood) there is nothing that can be done by first-aid. Beefsteak is useless for this purpose!

ALL BLACK EYES MUST BE SEEN SOON BY A DOCTOR TO EXCLUDE SERIOUS EYE INJURY OR A FRACTURE OF THE SKULL.

If there has been enough violence to cause a black eye there may also have been sufficient force to do serious injury to the eye or to cause a fracture of the skull.

9. *Internal bleeding following abdominal injury*

Place the casualty in a comfortable lying position, keep him at rest, and arrange for him to be taken swiftly to hospital. Write down the pulse rate and the time at five-minute intervals and continue to do this all the way to hospital.

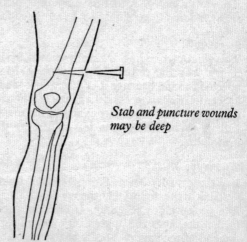

Stab and puncture wounds may be deep

A word of warning about certain kinds of wounds

Stab wounds and puncture wounds can cause serious deep injury or can be a method of planting infection deeply inside the body. The *skin* wound may be minor in such cases, but these injuries should always be regarded as serious – especially in the head and neck, around joints and near body cavities such as the chest or abdomen, and in the hand. Do not attempt home treatment in such cases. Apply first-aid and send the casualty to hospital.

Life-Saving First-Aid II

Summary of first-aid for BLEEDING

EXTERNAL BLEEDING

RECOGNIZE that BLEEDING is OCCURRING

STOP the BLEEDING

- PRESS where the blood is coming from
- ELEVATE arm or leg
- REST and continue to KEEP STILL to aid clot formation and stop clot breaking

BLEEDING CONTINUES→BLEEDING STOPS

- PRESS more firmly
- ELEVATE higher
- ADD dressings ON TOP of existing dressings and bandage more firmly

If blood loss has been other than very little, blood replacement may be needed. If bleeding has been moderate or severe, send quickly to hospital

This should stop the bleeding

SEND TO HOSPITAL

INTERNAL BLEEDING

RECOGNIZE that BLEEDING is OCCURRING
- pale colour, feeble pulse, clammy skin
- blood may be coughed or vomited, etc (visible internal bleeding)

REST the casualty
tell him to lie down and be still

SEND TO HOSPITAL
quickly if blood loss is due to internal bleeding

On the way to hospital

- Write down the pulse rate and the time at five-minute intervals. If the pulse rate rises, check that all sources of external bleeding have been stopped and look for bleeding underneath the casualty; if no external bleeding is found, the casualty must be bleeding intern-ally. If the pulse rate rises rapidly, get the casualty SWIFTLY to hospital

Chapter 5

UNCONSCIOUSNESS

Introduction

People frequently die following unconsciousness. They may need skilled help quickly if they are not to die. Priorities must be observed and the top priority is to preserve and maintain life (*see* Chapter 2). If the casualty is unconscious beware of wasting time by 'treating' trivial injuries.

Definition

Any departure whatever from the normal full alertness indicates some loss of consciousness. This can vary from inability to carry out intricate movements to being incapable of any response whatsoever. In this latter state, the casualty is incapable of self-preservation. If the casualty cannot speak to you coherently in sentences, he should always be treated as unconscious.

The AIMS of FIRST-AID for UNCONSCIOUSNESS are to:

Relieve and prevent obstructed breathing.
Send the casualty to hospital as soon as possible.

Any casualty who:
— is not fully alert
— cannot reply to questions in sentences (not words or grunts)

should be treated as an unconscious casualty.

How to treat any unconscious casualty (from whatever cause):
Relieve and prevent obstructed breathing.

   (i) Clear the mouth quickly of any debris, dentures, blood, vomit or loose natural teeth.

  (ii) Turn the casualty into the unconscious position with a slight head-down tip.

(i) Clear the mouth *quickly* of dentures, debris, blood, vomit or loose natural teeth. Any of these things can quite easily obstruct the air passage and cause obstructed breathing. Much can be removed by the careful use of the index finger; dentures, debris or loose natural teeth can quickly be picked out. A handkerchief or paper tissue can be a great help in removing blood or vomit.

An obstructed mouth often means that a casualty's feeble efforts to breathe are insufficient to maintain life; an *un*-obstructed mouth will allow the casualty to breathe and live.

(ii) Turn the casualty into the unconscious position with a slight head-down tip. All unconscious casualties left lying on their backs are in danger of obstructed breathing. This is due to the tongue falling to the back of the throat, or to blood or vomit (which is neither coughed out nor swallowed in the unconscious casualty). If vomiting occurs, as soon as the vomit reaches the throat it is likely to be breathed into the lungs. This will almost certainly cause a very severe pneumonia and possibly death.

It is interesting to note that the commonest cause of death in a casualty who has been unconscious following a head injury and who survives the immediate brain damage is pneumonia, caused by inhalation of saliva or vomit. *These deaths are completely preventable by you as a first-aider by the use of the unconscious position with a slight head-down tip.*

The easiest way to put someone into the unconscious position quickly is to place them in a face-down position, with the head turned towards the side on which you are standing. Then, all that is needed is three pulls: pull up the leg, pull up the arm and pull up the chin. The leg and arm are pulled up to act as props, thus preventing the casualty from flopping into a fully face-down position. Pulling up the chin maintains full neck extension in the teeth-clenched position and thus prevents obstructed breathing because the tongue is attached to the inside of the lower jaw. So remember the three pulls in placing a casualty into the unconscious position – leg, arm and chin!

Now arrange a slight head-down tip. Fluids drain downhill, so if a head-down tip is allied, any fluid in the air passages will tend to drain out through the mouth or nose and will thus be prevented from reaching the lungs. If the casualty is on a bed.

lift the foot of the bed and rest it on a chair.

If the casualty is on a stretcher, raise the foot of the stretcher by about one foot. Keep the head-down tip until the casualty reaches hospital.

The combination of the unconscious position and a slight head-down tip is life-saving. Unconscious casualties often vomit during recovery, and correct treatment will prevent the vomit from obstructing the air passages or from being inhaled, thus causing pneumonia. A pillow will tend to provide a 'head-up' tip and must, therefore, not be used.

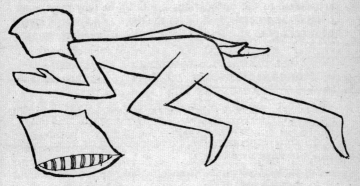

The unconscious position – do not use a pillow

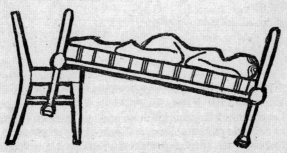

Lift the foot of the bed

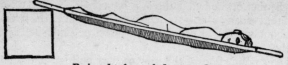

Raise the foot of the stretcher

Unconscious casualties must NEVER BE LEFT ALONE. They must be watched carefully to recognize any change in their condition which may require action on the part of the first-aider. For example, during recovery, some casualties become restless and excited (requiring gentle restraint and efforts to keep them in the unconscious position), or they may vomit. Should the general condition of the casualty get worse, it may be necessary to give artificial respiration if breathing stops.

ALL CASUALTIES WHO ARE OR HAVE BEEN UNCONSCIOUS MUST BE SENT TO HOSPITAL, OR MUST BE SEEN BY A DOCTOR

The main points in dealing with *any* unconscious casualty will therefore be:

   (i) clear the mouth *quickly* of dentures, debris, vomit, blood or loose natural teeth.

   (ii) turn casualty into the unconscious position with a slight head-down tip.

   (iii) loosen tight clothing at the neck and waist.

   (iv) send quickly to hospital, after ensuring that all serious injuries are treated.

— Look for bleeding, and stop any serious bleeding. Bleeding may not be obvious but it can be life-threatening (*see* Chapter 4, p 52).

— Fractures of limb bones should be immobilized. Transfer of the unconscious patient to hospital should not be delayed by treating trivialities, eg, abrasions or broken toes.

— Give nothing by mouth to unconscious casualties. The by-mouth rule in first-aid says: 'Give nothing by mouth except to conscious burned casualties or to conscious poisoned casualties.'

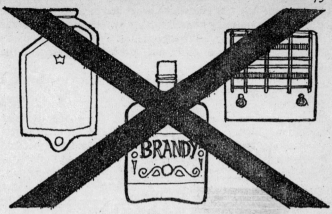

Nothing by mouth, do not heat, no alcohol

— Cover with one blanket only.

— Maintain a continuous watch on an unconscious casualty or one that has recently recovered – he may relapse. Never leave an unconscious casualty unattended. Do not attempt to rouse an unconscious casualty. Splashing their faces with water or slapping their cheeks is a waste of time and may even be dangerous.

Conclusion

The treatment of the unconscious casualty which is outlined above applies to unconsciousness from *any* cause. It is not the job of the first-aider to sort out the many different causes of unconsciousness – this is the doctor's task. But it *is* the duty of the first-aider to preserve life and to get the casualty to hospital without delay. This can be done by following the simple procedures outlined in this chapter on how to treat the unconscious casualty. **We believe that the correct treatment of unconsciousness has the largest life-saving potential of any first-aid procedure.**

Fits (*convulsions*)

Casualties with fits should be placed in the unconscious position, with a head-down tip if possible, and should be sent to hospital. Any restraint which is applied in order to stop the casualty from injuring himself further by the movements of the fit *must be gentle*; on no account use force. Move all hard objects such as chairs, table or other such articles out of range of the casualty's arms or legs.

Babies with fits are handled more easily when wrapped in a sheet or blanket.

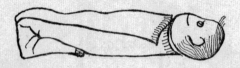

Wrap baby in a sheet or blanket

A WORD OF WARNING ABOUT ALCOHOL, INJURIES AND ILLNESS

Although there is a frequent connexion between drink and injuries, NEVER assume that because a casualty's breath smells of alcohol, he is drunk or under the influence of drink. A smell of alcohol in the breath means that drink has been taken: it does *not* tell how much alcohol has been consumed, nor does it mean that the condition of the casualty is *due* to alcohol intoxication.

Head injuries, bleeding, and some illnesses can produce alteration of consciousness, which closely resembles the results of alcohol intoxication.

ALWAYS assume that a casualty may have other injuries or may be ill until you have examined him carefully. Then, if you find no other reason for his condition, you should pass him on for further treatment. Alcohol in large doses is a poison and deaths have resulted from acute overdoses. Any casualty who has difficulty in walking and speaking may easily vomit and become unconscious, and will require appropriate treatment and careful watching in exactly the same way as any unconscious casualty.

Summary of first-aid for UNCONSCIOUSNESS

Life–Saving First Aid III

CHECK for BREATHING

Listen with ear over nose and mouth

Look at lower chest and upper abdomen for movement

→ **NOT BREATHING**

RELIEVE OBSTRUCTED BREATHING

Bend head back as far as it will go, and support lower jaw in teeth-clenched position. Quickly remove dentures, debris, loose natural teeth, blood and vomit from the mouth and throat

→ **NOT BREATHING**

Give artificial respiration (see summary of not breathing, page 51)

→ **BREATHING**

→ **BREATHING**

PREVENT OBSTRUCTED BREATHING

Quickly remove dentures, debris, loose natural teeth, blood and vomit from the mouth and throat

Place casualty in the **UNCONSCIOUS POSITION** with a slight head-down tip. Keep head bent back and lower jaw in teeth-clenched position

Check for other **SERIOUS INJURIES** and **TREAT** appropiately

Send the casualty to **HOSPITAL** as soon as possible

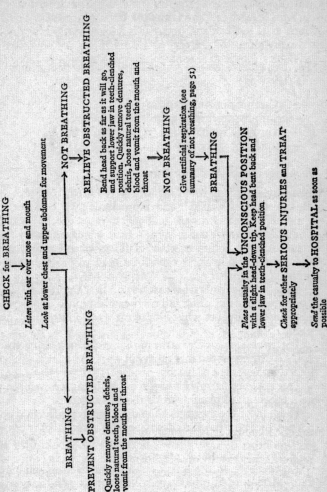

Chapter 6

BANDAGING

The aims of bandaging in first-aid will include one or more of the following:

- to keep a dressing in place;
- to apply pressure to a dressing or wound;
- to provide support;
- to prevent movement.

Improvised bandages and dressings

In many situations when first-aid is required, bandages and dressings are not available and improvisation will be necessary.

At home, sheets, towels and pillow-cases can be used for dressings or can be cut or torn to form bandages. Away from home, scarves, cotton or other clothing, clean handkerchiefs and paper handkerchiefs can all be used to provide wound-dressing materials.

Slings can be made from scarves and ties. Improvised slings can be made out of belts, and coats can be pinned or otherwise adapted to support wrists or arms (*see* illustration over page).

The *triangular bandage* is the most useful bandage in first-aid as it may be employed in a variety of ways – as a large sling, or folded into a broad or narrow bandage.

The broad or narrow bandages can be used, for example, to hold dressings in place or to tie the legs together.

The end of the bandage should be securely tied in a reef bow. A reef bow has the advantage over a knot that it can be easily untied, thus saving the casualty discomfort when the bandages are removed in hospital.

Tie the bow on the uninjured side, or over an uninjured limb. Make sure that the casualty is not resting on the bow, as this can be very unpleasant. Remember, an unconscious casualty cannot tell you that a bow (or knot) is pressing into him.

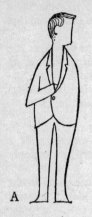

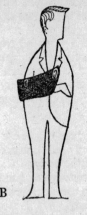

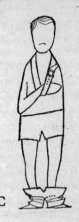

A

Arm inside coat

B

Coat flap pinned

C

Belt supporting arm

HOW TO FOLD A TRIANGULAR BANDAGE TO MAKE A BROAD OR A NARROW BANDAGE

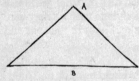

1. Fold A to B

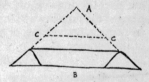

3. Now fold the top CC to B

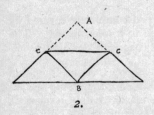

2.

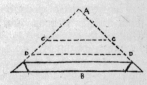

4. Fold the top of the broad bandage again to B. This makes a narrow bandage

The bandage should be tight enough to prevent movement of the injured part and to keep a dressing over a wound, but not so tight that it restricts circulation. After applying bandages always check the colour of the fingers or toes to make sure that there is no blueness (*see* page 107).

There will be occasions when no triangular bandages are available and improvisations are essential, for example by using scarves, ties, belts, folded handkerchiefs or similar items. Adhesive tape and cellulose tape may be very useful to fix dressings on regions which are difficult to bandage such as the face.

Roller bandaging

The usual prepared bandage is a gauze open-weave bandage which does not stretch and needs practice to learn how to apply it to the various parts of the body.

Crêpe, elasticated or conforming bandages are much better because they are easier to use, are less likely to loosen, and will apply pressure more evenly.

Begin bandaging limbs at the lowest point and work upwards – ie, begin nearest the fingers or toes and bandage towards the shoulder or hip. Start the bandage around the narrow part of a limb. First fix the bandage to the limb by overlapping the first few turns. Then gradually bandage upwards and over the dressing, overlapping each turn of bandage. Finish beyond the dressing by pinning the bandage with a safety-pin, by using adhesive tape, or by tying a reef knot in the split end of the bandage.

DRESSINGS

Prepared wound-dressings, often called field or mine dressings, will be found in most first-aid kits and are of different sizes, but are basically of the same design.

They consist of a cotton wool pad completely covered by plain absorbent gauze and stitched to a roller bandage. The whole is then wrapped in an outer cover and sterilized.

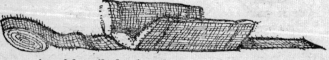

A useful sterile dressing, the prepared wound dressing

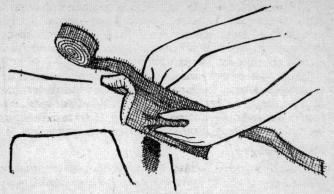

Apply the dressing to the wound without touching the inner sterile surface of the dressing pad

To apply this dressing:
— open the outer cover, usually by pulling a rip cord;
— remove any wrappings;
— unroll the short end of the roller bandage;
— grasp both ends of the bandage and pull open the dressing WITHOUT touching the inner surface of the dressing pad;
— quickly apply the pad to the wound;
— secure the dressing in place by holding the short end of the bandage and wrapping the long end around the limb. Finally tie the ends of the bandage together over the dressing in a reef bow or knot.

The dressing is sterilized. Make sure that you keep it free from germs, SO DO NOT:
— touch the inside of the dressing to be applied to the wound;
— breathe or cough on the dressing, or allow the casualty to do this.

Be as quick as you can and gentle at all times.

If no prepared dressings are available, improvised dressings will be needed. Use freshly laundered handkerchiefs, strips of sheets, pillow slips or tea towels or the cleanest suitable covering which is available.

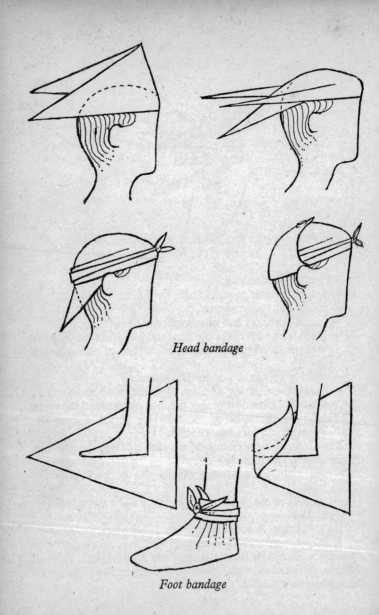

Head bandage

Foot bandage

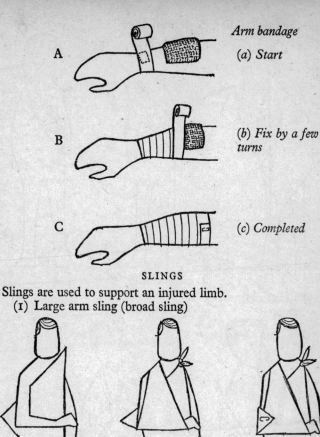

Arm bandage

A   (a) *Start*

B   (b) *Fix by a few turns*

C   (c) *Completed*

SLINGS

Slings are used to support an injured limb.

(1) Large arm sling (broad sling)

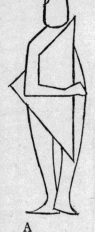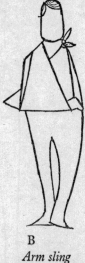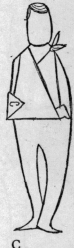

A   B   C

Arm sling

(2) Triangular sling (St John sling)

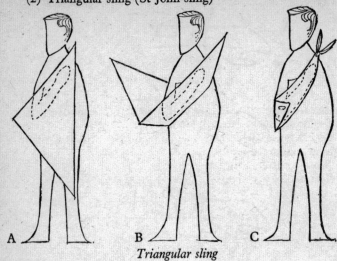

A   B   C

Triangular sling

(3) Collar and cuff

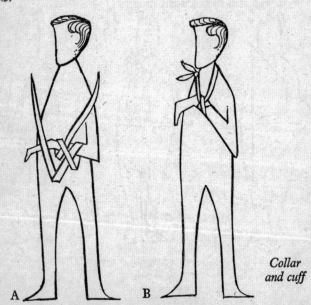

A   B

*Collar
and cuff*

Chapter 7

BURNS

Burns are injuries caused by heat, friction or chemicals.

Scalds are burns caused by hot liquids.

Severe burns affect the whole body, not just the part which can be seen to be burnt.

Most burns are PREVENTABLE.

The majority of burns occur in the home.

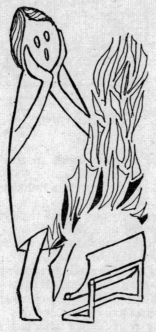

A common cause of burning

If anyone's clothing catches fire, much more of the body will be burned if the person is allowed to stand or run about than if they are *made* to lie down.

So, if you see anyone with clothes on fire, force them to lie down at once and then try to smother the flames, using a rug, blanket, carpet or coat. Be careful however that you do not get burned. The casualty depends on you. Then start cooling the burned areas *at once* (*see* page 90).

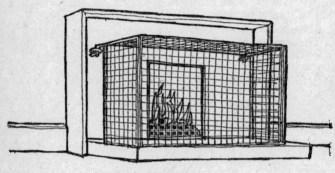

Guard all fires

Over one third of the casualties are children with burns caused mostly by burning clothing.

It is much easier to prevent a burn than to treat it. Guard all fires.

First-aid comes a very poor second to prevention.

Burns are classified as *superficial* or *deep* depending upon whether the burn penetrates shallowly or deeply, resulting in partial or complete skin loss.

The severity of a burn depends on a combination of factors, but THE BEST GUIDE TO SEVERITY IN FIRST-AID IS THE AREA OF THE BURN. Small deep burns are much less serious than large-area superficial burns.

The emergency treatment of a major burn is a life or death procedure.

Skin loss needs skin replacement in hospital.

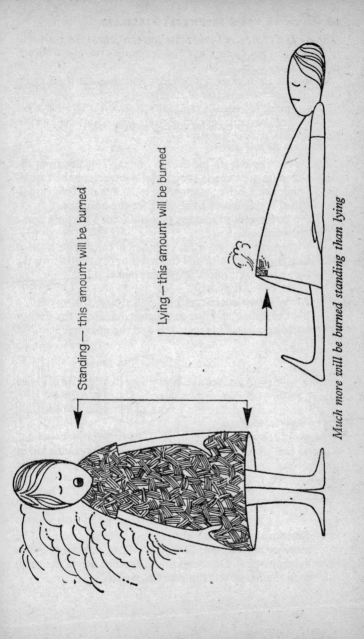

Standing — this amount will be burned

Lying — this amount will be burned

Much more will be burned standing than lying

The AIMS of FIRST-AID for BURNS are to:

1. Prevent further damage.
2. Prevent infection.
3. Minimize the effects of loss of fluid from the burned tissues.
4. Reassure the burned person.
5. Transport the casualty swiftly to hospital.

1. *Prevent further damage*

Remove the cause from the casualty or the casualty from the cause. If there are experts present let them rescue the casualties. Think twice before attempting to be a hero. Two casualties instead of one makes more work for the hospitals.

If you do attempt to rescue a casualty from a burning house or other building:

— Remember that smoke is responsible for more deaths at fires than actual heat and that a wet or dry cloth across the face will NOT protect you from smoke.
— Wear gloves if possible.
— Always open doors carefully. When a door is opened, a blast of hot air and flame may rush out. Keep the door or an adjacent wall between you and the opening.

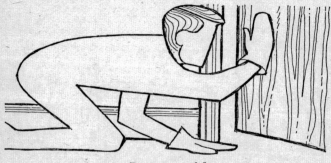

Be very careful

— Crawl on your stomach if possible because there will be more air at ground or floor level. When searching, follow a definite plan. Go round the walls, then across the room with the hands searching at full stretch.

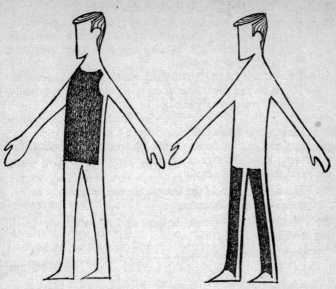

Adults with burns of this much or more of the body surface need transfusion in hospital

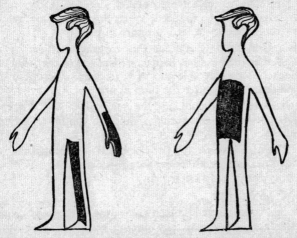

Children with burns of this much or more of the body surface need transfusion in hospital

— Remember to search the cupboards, wardrobes and under beds – people may go to these places to escape from heat. Feel on the bed – the casualty may have been overcome by smoke while sleeping.

— Do not delay – get the casualty out as quickly as possible.

— If you do not know how to carry an unconscious casualty on your own you should not be in there.

— Above all do not panic if you feel you have lost your way – find your way around the walls to the door.

(a) *Heat and friction burns* should be treated *immediately* by showering in cold water or by immersion in water which is cooler than body temperature.

The aim is to *cool* the burned areas as quickly as possible after burning.

This cooling process should be kept up for ten minutes in all but trivial burns.

The effect of this treatment is twofold:

(i) *Cooling* – this lessens the severity of the burn and thus aids subsequent hospital treatment;

(ii) *Relief of pain* – burns are often very painful, and cooling relieves pain. Cooling should be continued for ten minutes or for a longer period, until no further relief from pain is produced by cooling or withdrawal of cooling does not lead to return of pain.

It is important to carry out this treatment *as quickly as possible* after the burn has happened. Use the nearest cold tap or bucket. A considerable part of burn damage occurs in the period immediately after the burn injury.

(b) *Chemical burns* should have the chemical washed off *at once* in tap or shower. Showering should be continued for ten minutes.

The aim is to *remove* the chemical at once so that it does not produce further injury and to *dilute* any remaining chemical.

2. *Prevent infection*

The skin is the normal protective covering of the body. When the skin has been destroyed by burning, germs are able to enter and multiply rapidly in the tissue fluid and damaged tissue.

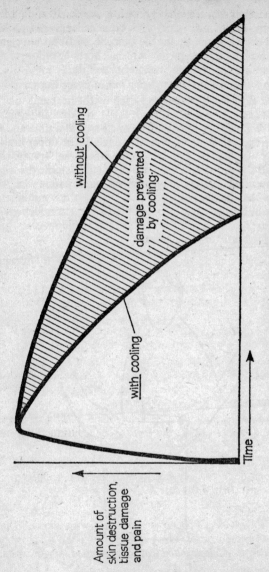

Cooling burns and scalds prevents damage and pain

Cover the burned area quickly with a sterile dressing large enough to cover *more* than the burned area. Pre-packed sterilized dressings are by far the best. Second-best are clean, unused and well-ironed handkerchiefs, sheets or pillow-cases. Any smooth, clean, *non-fluffy* material will do.

DO NOT use *cotton-wool* or *hairy lint* to cover burns.

Burned clothes are usually sterilized by the heat and stick to the skin – *leave them in place.* Place the sterile dressing quickly over the clothes. Try to cover one small area at a time and fix the covering, rather than doing all at once. If the upper limb is burned, cover first the hand, then the wrist, the forearm, the elbow and the upper arm each with a separate sterile dressing. This allows the dressings to be taken off one at a time when the dressings are being replaced in hospital, thus minimizing exposure of burned areas and helping to prevent infection.

At home, clean, freshly ironed sheets or pillow-cases may be used for burns of large areas.

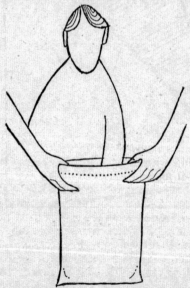

A clean pillow-case may be used

Pillow-slips can be used to encase the forearm and hand or foot – and a bolster-slip may take an arm or leg. Place the limb inside the pillow-slip, apply some padding outside, and then bandage the padding over the pillow-case. Use an arm sling to keep the arm at rest. Burn dressings should always be padded or have several layers of dressing materials applied in order to absorb any leakage of fluid which may seep through from the burned area.

DO NOT burst or break blisters.

DO NOT apply any lotion, grease or antiseptic.

DO NOT cough or breathe over the burned area.

DO NOT touch the burned area. Hands are always covered with germs.

DO NOT undress and handle the casualty or the burned areas more than is necessary.

DO NOT take the dressing off again.

DO NOT apply cotton-wool, fluffy or hairy materials to burned areas.

Scarring is a late complication of burns, but serious in that it causes disfigurement. Help to reduce scarring by keeping germs out.

3. *Minimize the effects of loss of fluid from the burned tissues*

When skin is damaged the body is not able to retain the body fluids which are part of every tissue. This fluid leaks out as a straw-coloured, slightly sticky fluid, from the burned areas, and may form blisters or leak away, depending on the severity of the burn. It may, however, be discoloured by the charred tissues. In burns of large areas, the volume of fluid lost soon becomes serious. Conscious burned *adult* casualties should be given drinks of water, weak tea or milk (but not alcohol) in quantities of about half a cupful every ten minutes until they get to hospital. Larger amounts than this may cause vomiting. This treatment will help the casualty to resist the effects of burning and will make hospital treatment more effective. Remember, NO fluids by mouth may be given to an unconscious casualty; you may kill him.

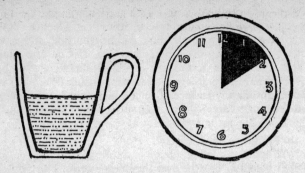

4. *Reassure the burned person*

You must remain calm and by example bring fresh hope. Make the casualty as comfortable as possible. An injured person is frightened – a burned person is terrified. He is thinking 'What has happened – am I going to live, am I scarred and disfigured for life ?' Relieve his anxiety and tell him he is in good hands.

5. *Transport the casualty swiftly to hospital*

Remember to give the casualty half a cup of water every ten minutes during his journey to hospital.

Superficial (surface) burns are usually very painful. Deep burns often are not, because the nerves which carry the sensation of pain have been destroyed.

Because burns are often followed by swelling of the burned part, any constriction such as a ring or bracelet should be removed at once.

If there are a number of burn casualties, the ones with the largest area of burn should be sent to hospital first.

Some examples of first-aid for burns

1. *Heat burns*

— cool at once by showering or by immersion in cold water;
— cover the burned area (and burned clothes) with sterile dressings or with the cleanest available covering;
— lay the casualty down;

— if there is a large-area burn on a limb, immobilize the limb as if it were fractured;

— give the casualty, if conscious, half a cupful of water or other bland fluid every ten minutes;

— send him to hospital without delay.

Heat burns from a nuclear explosion may be due to heat flash or to secondary fires. They may be surface burns or deep burns. The treatment is the same as for any other burn.

2. *Scalds*

Cool at once by showering or by immersion in cold water. If the clothes are soaked and not stuck to the skin, remove the clothes. Then treat as a heat burn.

3. *Chemical burns*

Serious burns can be caused by chemicals such as:

(*a*) Acids – sulphuric, hydrochloric, nitric, glacial acetic, etc.

(*b*) Alkalis – caustic soda, caustic potash, quicklime, ammonia, etc.

Acids or alkalis are often called 'corrosive liquids'.

The AIMS of FIRST-AID for CHEMICAL BURNS are to:

Remove the chemical by washing or showering, thus preventing further damage.

Treat as a heat burn.

REMOVE THE CHEMICAL

Immediate removal prevents the chemical from continuing to cause further damage to the skin; speed is essential. The sooner and the more efficiently the chemical is removed, the less will be the resultant burn.

TIME SPENT ON ADEQUATE AND CAREFUL REMOVAL OF CHEMICALS IS TIME WELL SPENT, AND THIS PART OF THE TREATMENT SHOULD NOT BE SKIMPED OR HURRIED. Removal should be thought of *first* as a process of getting rid of the chemical by flushing it off (ie, a mechanical removal of chemical) and *second* as dilution. Use *large amounts of* water.

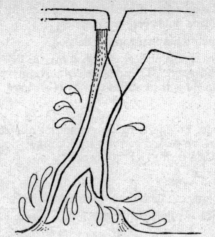

Use large amounts of water for chemical burns

(i) Quickly start washing the affected area with running water from a tap or shower. This washes off and dilutes the chemical whether it is acid or alkali.
(ii) Remove all contaminated clothing during washing.
(iii) Continue washing until all the chemical has been re-moved. TEN MINUTES washing, timed by the clock, will usually be required.

THEN TREAT AS A HEAT BURN

(i) Dry sterile padded dressing.
(ii) Fluids by mouth, half a cupful every ten minutes, if conscious.
(iii) To hospital without delay.

Chemical burns of the eye

These cause great pain. Start treatment IMMEDIATELY. This can save scarring of the eye and possible loss of vision.

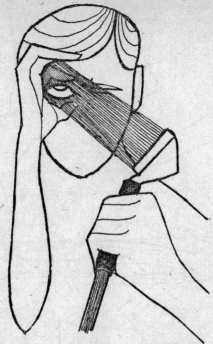

Wash well with water – self-help

(i) Turn the head towards the affected side to prevent fluid pouring into the good eye.

(ii) Irrigate the eye with copious amounts of running tap-water. Separate the eyelids with your fingers so that the water can wash the chemical away from the inside of the lids and from the eyeball. Continue for 10–15 minutes *by the clock*. DO NOT SKIMP OR HURRY THIS STEP.

(iii) Now cover gently with a sterile pad and bandage.

(iv) Send the casualty to hospital as soon as possible.

4. *Electrical burns*

An electric shock may stop the casualty from breathing, and will often cause small deep burns.

T–D

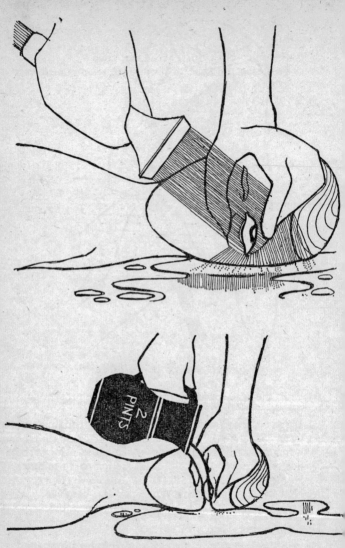

Wash well holding the eyelids apart – first-help

The *AIMS* of *FIRST-AID* for *ELECTROCUTION* are to:

Have the source of electricity switched off.
Check breathing and apply artificial respiration immediately if not breathing.
Treat any burns.

HAVE THE SOURCE OF ELECTRICITY TURNED OFF

Make sure it is safe to approach the casualty. Try to have the electrical supply disconnected. In the home, switch off the current and remove the plug. Pull the insulated wire to remove a live appliance from the casualty if you cannot switch off.

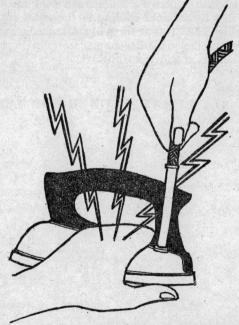

If you cannot switch off, pull on the insulated wire

When all else fails ease the casualty from the electricity supply with an insulated lever. Remember that water is a good conductor of electricity so use only dry material and keep out of any liquids in which the casualty may be lying.

CHECK BREATHING

Establish whether breathing is present. If not, start artificial respiration immediately. It may be necessary to continue this for a prolonged period (*see* Chapter 3).

TREAT AS A HEAT BURN (*see* page 91)

The importance of cooling burns

Recent research, reported at an international burns congress, showed that **immediate cooling is the most important thing which can be done for a burn.** Immediate cooling is probably more important than hospital treatment in preventing loss of life, loss of skin or scarring.

Remember –
COOL ALL BURNS AT ONCE FOR TEN MINUTES

Summary of first-aid for BURNS

Heat burns and scalds

1. Cool immediately → Put casualty in a cool shower or bath, or put the burned part under a running tap of cold water or in a basinful of cold water. Remove clothing unless it is stuck to the skin

2. Continue cooling for 10 minutes → Do not skimp or hurry this step

3. Cover the burned areas and adjacent skin → Use a sterile dressing, if possible, or the cleanest, *non-fluffy* cover available

4. Replace fluids → If casualty is conscious, give sips of water every ten minutes (*see* page 93 for quantities). Give nothing by mouth to unconscious casualties

5. Send to hospital → Give *sips* of water every 10 minutes

Chemical burns

1. Remove the chemical AT ONCE → Wash *at once* with large amounts of running water from a tap, shower, hose or spray. Remove clothing which may have chemical on it. Give prior and special attention to the eyes, holding the lids apart to let water in

2. Continue flushing with water for 10 minutes → Do not skimp or hurry this step. The chemical must be adequately removed

3. Continue as indicated under heat burns, 3

Continued on next page

Electrical Burns

1. Make sure that the ELECTRICITY IS OFF ⟶ Do not become the next casualty yourself
   before going near the casualty

2. When the electricity is off, approach and
   LISTEN for BREATHING

   Breathing   Not breathing ⟶ If breathing has stopped, give artificial respiration (*see page 44*)

3. Check for unconsciousness

   Conscious   Unconscious ⟶ If unconscious, place in the unconscious position

4. Continue as indicated under heat burns, I

   If more than half an hour has passed ⟶ Omit cooling, cover all burns, and send quickly to hospital
   since burning or if breathing has
   stopped, or if the casualty has been or
   is unconscious

Chapter 8

FRACTURES AND DISLOCATIONS

A fracture is a broken or cracked bone. There are two sorts of fractures, closed and open.

1. A CLOSED fracture has no wound at or near it.
2. An OPEN fracture has a wound at or near it.

1. CLOSED fractures are more common and may be serious or not serious depending on the amount of damage around the ends of the broken bone, and the amount of blood which escapes into the tissues. The bone may be broken into two or more pieces, but all these pieces are covered by unbroken skin.

2. OPEN fractures have a wound leading down to the site of the fracture. The bone may protrude from this wound. The wound may be a very small one and may even appear to be closed over. If, however, an open fracture is suspected – TREAT IT AS OPEN. A wound allows germs to cause infection of the bone and infection will delay healing. An open fracture is, therefore, a fracture plus a wound.

How to tell if there is a fracture (diagnosis)

An X-ray picture taken in hospital may be the only *sure* way of knowing that a bone is broken. However, where any part of the body has been subjected to a heavy blow or other force, and the part is mis-shapen (deformity), is swollen (blood lost from the circulation), and the casualty cannot use the part normally (loss of function), it can safely be assumed that the bone is broken.

A more detailed list of facts which may be used in deciding about fractures is given below:

HISTORY – A casualty may describe receiving a heavy blow, perhaps feeling something give way or snap, followed by severe pain and being unable to use his limb, or whatever part is injured.

PAIN – is usually severe and may even cause the casualty to shout. It is present near the site of the fracture and is made worse when the injured part is moved.

TENDERNESS – may be felt over the fracture site by light touch during examination of the casualty. Be gentle.

DEFORMITY – may be more obvious when compared with the other side. Always remember to compare the injured with the uninjured side. A limb may be bent or twisted into an unusual position or even shortened.

SWELLING – (which is due to loss of blood into the tissues) may occur, together with discoloration or bruising. This does not provide reliable evidence of fracture. The swelling may be so marked as to prevent accurate assessment of any injury to deeper parts. If in doubt always assume that a fracture is present.

IRREGULARITY – can often be seen in an open fracture. In a closed fracture the sharp edges of the broken bones or a gap between the broken ends may be felt.

LOSS OF USE – of the injured part may be obvious, but if the ends of the bones have been forced into each other, the casualty may be able to use the limb, even though it is fractured.

UNNATURAL MOVEMENT – at the site of the fracture may be felt and at the same time a feeling of grating (crepitus) may be noted. The limb feels limp and wobbly. Unnatural movement should never be produced deliberately as this may worsen the injury. However, if you do notice unnatural movement, maintain your grasp and support the part to prevent further injury. Unnatural movement means that the fracture is unstable and is likely to become open – so handle such injuries with extra care.

The *AIMS* of *FIRST-AID* for *FRACTURES* are to:

Cover all *open* fractures (stop bleeding, prevent infection).

Prevent further damage by stopping movement from occurring round the break (that is, immobilize the fracture).
Send the casualty to hospital.

COVER ALL OPEN FRACTURES

(i) *Treat the wound* – stop severe bleeding. Cover the wound with a sterile dressing to prevent infection. Build up dressings around the wound so that no pressure is applied on the broken ends of the bone. (*See* Chapter 4, page 63.) Do not attempt to replace protruding bone ends.

(ii) *Treat the fracture* – once the wound has been treated, the treatment of both open and closed fractures then follows the same principles.

PREVENT FURTHER DAMAGE BY IMMOBILIZING THE FRACTURE

Simple immobilization prevents further injury and promotes the comfort of the casualty. If the surroundings make it safe to do so, it is usually best to immobilize the fracture *before* moving the casualty.

SEND THE CASUALTY TO HOSPITAL

All fractures or doubtful fractures *have* to be X-rayed and hospital treatment is essential. Any fractures may give rise to blood loss from the circulation due to internal bleeding, and in the case of fracture of large bones or of multiple fractures, this blood loss may require blood replacement soon.

Some general points concerning the first-aid treatment of fractures

— Do not attempt to straighten limbs: leave this to the hospital. It is far better to immobilize the limb in the position in which you find it, if it is comfortable, than to move it forcibly.

— If it is necessary to move an injured limb which is broken, apply gentle but firm traction. This means trying to pull the limb slowly, gently but firmly away from the body by pulling on the casualty's hand or foot. Do not relax your traction until the limb is secured. To do so causes great pain.

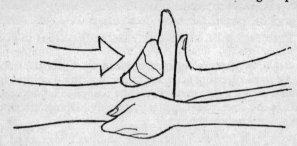

Pull gently but firmly

— Usually, the best way to stop movement from occurring in the arm is to fix it to the trunk. An injured leg should be tied to the opposite leg. Artificial rigid support by splints is needed only when both the legs are broken.

— In limbs, the site of the fracture together with the joint above and the joint below should all be immobilized.

— Use plenty of padding to fill in all the natural hollows before bandaging arm to body or leg to leg. Use padding to cover bony points such as the inner side of the elbows, knees and ankles. This makes the casualty more comfortable and stops him fidgeting, which will cause more pain.

— *Fractures are a cause of internal bleeding*. This bleeding takes place from the blood vessels inside the broken bone, from the blood vessels encircling the broken bone and from the damaged tissues around the fracture. As much as a pint of blood may be lost from the circulation even from small breaks in bones.

From a fracture of the shin bone two pints of blood may be lost from the circulation and give rise to swelling. Bleeding caused by a fractured thigh bone may amount to as much as four pints of blood lost into the tissues. Any casualty who has a fracture of a large bone such as the thigh bone, or who has several fractures, may be suffering from blood loss from the circulation due to internal bleeding. Severe bleeding needs urgent treatment (*see* Chapter 4, page 55). Blood loss needs blood replacement SOON. Therefore, casualties who have fractures of large bones or who have multiple fractures must be sent quickly to hospital after the essential treatment has been carried out.

— There is usually no need for elborate bandaging in a conscious casualty. Emergency treatment must be simple, neat and an effective preliminary to hospital treatment.

— First-aid must not delay hospital treatment. Do not waste time treating trivialities. Send the casualty to hospital for further treatment as soon as possible.

— When using bandages to immobilize fractures, tie *reef* bows (or *reef* knots) very firmly. The bow (or knot) should be tied away from a known site of injury – for example over the uninjured leg when tying legs together. Bows are easier to undo than knots, and, properly tied, with the ends out of the way, should be as secure as knots.

— *Always look for any signs which indicate that the circulation in a limb is becoming impaired* by swelling, deformity or tight dressings, both before and after carrying out first-aid treat-treatment. Look for:

   (i) blue or white extremities (fingers and toes) or any change from the normal pink colour.

  (ii) loss of feeling below the injury. Test by asking the casualty if he can feel you lightly touching his fingertips and toes.

 (iii) no pulse at the wrist or ankle.

If there is any doubt about circulation, loosen all tight dressings and straighten out the limb. BENT ELBOWS ARE SPECIALLY DANGEROUS IN CHILDREN WHO HAVE FRACTURES OR DISLOCATIONS NEAR THE ELBOW. Tell the doctor immediately after you get to hospital about any troubles with circulation which you have observed.

IF THERE IS ANY DOUBT AT ALL *whether there is or is not a fracture*, ALWAYS TREAT AS A FRACTURE.

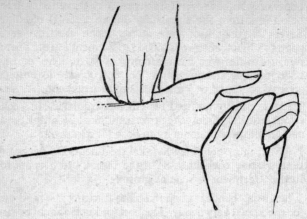

Taking the pulse – this needs practice

Detailed examples of fracture treatment will be given under the following headings:

1. Upper limb
2. Lower limb
3. Nose and jaw
4. Spine
5. Pelvis
6. Chest and ribs

I. UPPER LIMB

A. *Collar bone, shoulder blade and shoulder*

The casualty will often clasp his arm against his chest or support the point of the elbow.

He usually complains of pain at the site of the fracture which becomes worse when the arm moves.

This group of fractures is often caused by falls on to the outstretched hand or on to the side with the arm underneath. The muscles of the region will usually immobilize the fracture sufficiently and emergency treatment is, therefore, simple.

(i) Place *loose* padding (about the size of your fist) in the armpit.

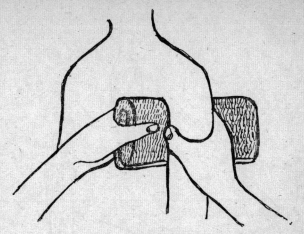

Place loose padding in the armpit

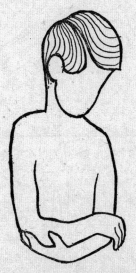

The good-arm sling

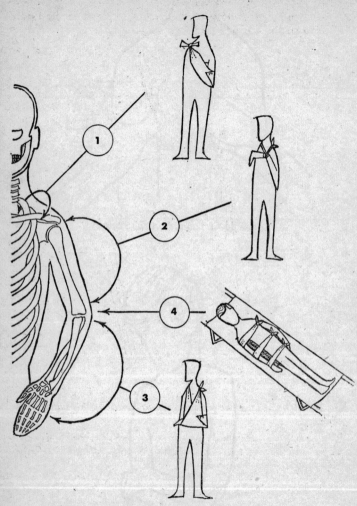

How to treat upper-limb fractures

(ii) Apply a triangular sling (St John sling).

(iii) Send him to hospital in a sitting position in the first available car or ambulance.

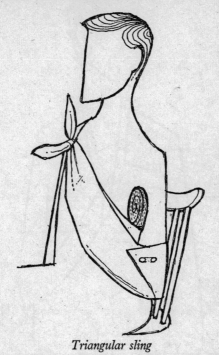

Triangular sling

B. *Arm: from just below the shoulder down to, and including, the elbow*

The casualty usually holds his arm to his chest and is frightened to let you touch him. The weight of the arm and forearm provides adequate traction.

Treatment

(i) *fractures of the upper and middle part of the arm bone*

Slowly bend the elbow, holding the wrist only, and place the fingertips of the injured side hand near the tip of the opposite shoulder. Apply a collar and cuff. Send him to hospital in *sitting* position in the first available car or ambulance.

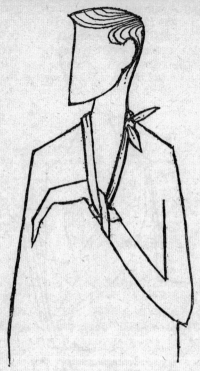

Collar and cuff

(ii) *fractures of the lower part of the arm bone and elbow region*

In fractures of this region, especially in children, there is considerable danger to the circulation below the injury. The artery which supplies blood to the forearm and hand lies very close to the lower end of the arm bone and this artery may be damaged by a jagged bone end or compressed by the swelling which occurs round the site of injury. Compression and direct injury to the artery may both occur. Any bending of the elbow may further directly damage the artery or cause increased compression, thus preventing blood from reaching the forearm and hand. Therefore, fractures near the elbow should be treated by fixing the limb to the trunk in a very slightly bent or near straight position. Place plenty of loose padding between the arm and the trunk. Secure the arm to the trunk with one broad bandage at the wrist and another just above the elbow swelling. Fix the forearm also if this will make the casualty more comfortable. Check the circulation (*see* page 107) especially in children. Transport to hospital as a stretcher case.

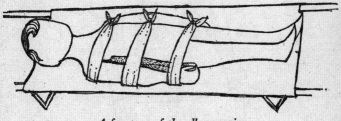

A fracture of the elbow region

An alternative method of first-aid for elbow-region injuries is to get the casualty to lie down and to place the injured arm gently on to one or several pillows, with the arm by the side and the hand in a palm-up position.

C. *The forearm (from just below the elbow), wrist, hand and fingers*

Fracture of the wrist is a very common injury, especially in elderly people, following a fall. The hand is put out to prevent the fall, and the wrist is injured.

In the forearm and wrist there is usually a lot of swelling, but the initial pain gradually subsides unless the limb is carelessly handled.

Treatment

Bend the limb at the elbow until the forearm lies across the body. Apply an arm sling (*see* page 83-4). Transport to hospital in a sitting position in the first available car or ambulance.

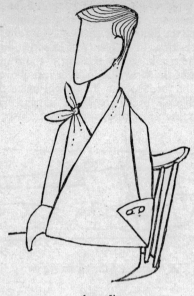

Arm sling

2. FRACTURES OF THE LOWER LIMB

A. *From hip to knee*

This is a serious injury. Send immediately for the ambulance. Up to four pints of blood may be lost from the circulation into the tissues around the fracture. This needs replacement by blood transfusion – the earlier the better – in hospital.

Treatment

(*a*) Fill the natural hollows of the body with ample loose padding.

  (i) Place a small pillow or the equivalent amount of padding between the thighs.

  (ii) Apply padding between the knees and ankles to prevent

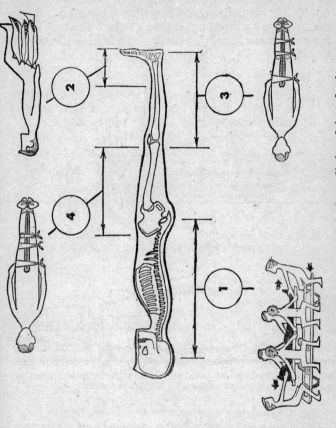

How to treat fractures of the lower limb, pelvis and spine

pain from pressure of these bony projections on each other.

(b) Bring the sound uninjured limb to the injured one. Make all limb movements carefully and slowly. Watch the casualty closely. He will tell you, or wince if he is being hurt. *Do not rush* 'because it will all be over more quickly'. This only causes further pain and injury. Support the foot firmly – do not let it flop about.

(c) Immobilize:

    (i) Tie both feet and ankles together with a broad bandage in a figure of eight. Leave the boots or shoes *on*, they make bandaging more effective and comfortable.

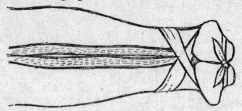

A figure-of-eight bandage round the feet and ankles

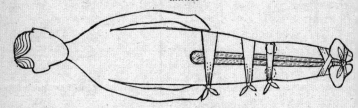

Bandage above and below the fracture

    (ii) Tie the knees together with a broad bandage.
    (iii) Tie a broad bandage both above and below the fracture.

Make sure that the bandages are neat. Tie the reef bows very firmly on the outside of the uninjured limb. If swelling continues, loosen the bandages so that they give support but do not obstruct the circulation.

(*d*) Send the casualty to hospital on a stretcher as soon as possible.

B. *From knee to foot*

A fracture of the leg is nearly as serious as a fracture of the thigh. Bleeding takes place in the region of the fracture from the broken bone and from the damaged muscles. As much as two pints of blood may be lost from the circulation. Blood loss needs blood replacement, in hospital, the earlier the better.

The shin bone lies just underneath the skin. A fracture of the shin bone, therefore, is very often an open fracture. If it is a closed fracture it can quite easily become an open fracture. Handle it with great care. All 'sprained' ankles should be treated as fractures until proved otherwise by X-ray.

Treatment

(*a*) Place adequate padding in the natural hollows.
  (i) Pad well between the thighs.
  (ii) Pad well between knees and ankles to prevent pressure pain.

(*b*) Bring the good leg to the injured leg (not the injured leg to the good leg). Support the foot of the injured limb firmly and apply slight traction. Careful, slow movements are of great importance in preventing pain and further damage.

(*c*) Immobilize:
  (i) Tie both feet and ankles together by means of a figure-of-eight bandage. Leave the shoes on. If the fracture is near the ankle simply tie the feet together.
  (ii) Tie the knees together with a broad bandage.
  (iii) Secure the fracture by tying a broad bandage both above and below the fracture.

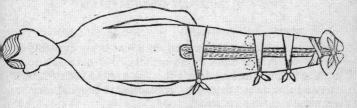

Fracture of the leg

If the fracture site is high or low on the leg, one of these bandages may have to be omitted so that pressure is not applied to the fracture by bandaging right over the site of the fracture.

(*d*) Send the casualty to hospital on a stretcher.

C. *Feet and toes*

Fracture of the small bones of the foot or toe can be satisfactorily treated as follows:

   (i) Leave the shoe on.
   (ii) Loosen and remove the laces.

This is a fracture which needs no treatment other than keeping the weight off the foot.

   (iii) Send to hospital as a sitting or stretcher case, but do not allow the casualty to bear weight on his feet. Being a hero usually makes the fracture worse!

Fractures of the ankle or of the feet and toes can often be very satisfactorily treated by resting the injured leg on a cushion or pillow, and by tying the cushion lightly on to the limb.

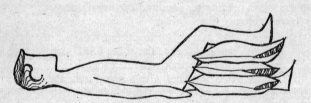

Pillows may be sufficient for a fractured ankle

D. *Fracture of both lower limbs*

An uninjured leg to use as a natural splint is not available in this severe injury. Send for an ambulance at once. There is usually severe bleeding inside the legs around each fracture site and this means that blood transfusion in hospital may be required as soon as possible.

Careful handling and some traction is essential.

Treatment

(*a*) Fill the natural hollows with ample padding.
   (i) Pad well between thighs.
   (ii) Pad well between knees and ankles.

(*b*) Very carefully, with traction, bring each leg in turn to approximately its normal position. Do not let the legs wag or fall. A temporary figure-of-eight bandage round the feet and ankles may help at this stage.

(*c*) If two long splints are available, pad them well and place one each side of the limbs from the armpits to just beyond the feet.

(*d*) Immobilize the limbs using the splints available. Extra support can be given by placing coats or blankets along each side of the limbs and feet to prevent side-to-side movement.

(*e*) Send the casualty to hospital as a stretcher case as soon as possible. If no long splints are available, user a shorter splint placed between the limbs from crutch to feet. If no splints are available, bandage the legs to each other and tie the reef bows firmly on the side showing the least injury, away from known injured areas.

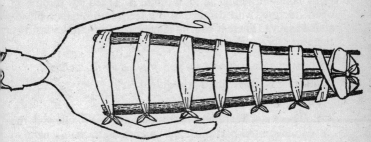

Fracture of both lower limbs

To avoid moving the injured limbs unnecessarily, pass the bandages under the natural hollows of the body – these are:

1. The neck.
2. The small of the back.
3. Just below the buttocks.
4. The hollow behind the knees.
5. Behind the ankles.

Then pass the bandage up or down gently into the required position.

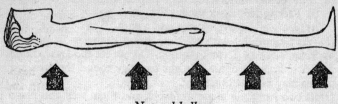

Natural hollows

3. THE NOSE AND JAW

Nose

This fracture is usually associated with bleeding from the nose which is discussed in Chapter 4, page 65.

Lower jaw

Fracture of the jaw is often caused by a severe blow on the chin – by hitting the windscreen of a car, or being hit by a fist, or by falling headlong on to the chin. A broken jaw is often an open fracture, with damage to the teeth and obvious blood-stained saliva. There is pain on moving the jaw and the casualty therefore speaks through clenched teeth.

The jaw muscles will hold the jaw in place by themselves.

Bandaging is, therefore, not required.

First-aid is necessary only if:

1. There is a fracture of both sides of the jaw, allowing the front central part of the jaw with the attached tongue to pass backwards and obstruct the airway.

2. A blood vessel in the tongue or cheek has been damaged.

The treatment of a fractured jaw is therefore:

(*a*) Maintain a free airway. Self-help may be applied by hooking the index fingers over and behind the lower front teeth and then pulling in a forward direction. If it is necessary, grasp the tongue with a handkerchief, and pull it forwards.

(b) Stop any serious bleeding.

(c) Send to hospital.

If the casualty is conscious, send him to hospital in the sitting position, leaning forwards, in the first available car or ambulance, with a receptacle for bloodstained saliva or vomit.

If the casualty is unconscious, send him – as any unconscious casualty – in the unconscious position with a slight head-down tip. Make sure that the jaw is pulled well forward and watch carefully for any sign of obstructed breathing.

4. SPINE OR BACKBONE

A fracture of the spine is a very serious injury.
It is commonly caused by:

(i) High divers plunging into a shallow pool.

(ii) A fall from a great height as in climbing, with the casualty landing on his back, feet or buttocks.

(iii) A heavy weight falling on to the back of the casualty.

(iv) Whiplash movement of the neck in a head-on or rear-end collision.

(v) Falls from a motor-cycle at speed.

The spine normally protects the enclosed spinal cord from damage. When the spine is broken this protection is lost and any careless movement may squeeze or sever the spinal cord. This results in permanent loss of movement (paralysis) and loss of feeling. The spinal cord once damaged will not grow again or recover.

Treat the casualty very carefully. Do not move him more than is essential.

How to diagnose a fractured spine

The casualty will usually be pale, anxious and complaining of pain at the site of the fracture. However, in some cases the casualty may appear tranquil and relatively free of pain following one of the types of injury listed in i–v above. Spinal injury should always be suspected following such causes.

If the spinal cord is damaged at the neck all four limbs may be paralysed (unable to be moved). The casualty may also find difficulty in breathing. If the spinal cord is damaged in the small of the back only the lower limbs may be paralysed. The casualty may also lose control of his bladder and bowel actions.

Test for loss of power and feeling by asking the casualty to move his big toes and fingers. He cannot move paralysed limbs. Touch or lightly pinch the skin of his ankles and hands. If the limbs are paralysed he will feel nothing. Do not expect to find a large swelling at the site of a fractured spine – there may be no swelling at all.

Occasionally, with severe spinal damage, the casualty may be unconscious.

A FRACTURED SPINE is an injury when SPEED in treatment is UNIMPORTANT. Take your time and prevent further damage. If you suspect a fractured spine first tell the casualty to lie still, then send for a doctor and an ambulance. Do not move the casualty in any way whatever until you are ready to move him properly as described below. The casualty must be carefully lifted on to a stretcher. He MUST be kept stiff and straight. All bending and twisting must be prevented. If he is allowed to bend forward and jack-knife he may die or suffer permanent paralysis, and loss of feeling.

Treatment

Warn the casualty to lie still. *Send for help*.

It should be emphasized that a casualty with a fracture (or suspected fracture) of the spine cannot be moved safely without several helpers – we would suggest a minimum of four people. Care in lifting and moving such casualties can make the difference between full recovery and lifelong paralysis of the legs. So, make sure before attempting to move such casualties that you take your time, that you make gentle but firm movements, and that you have enough helpers. Until you are sure that you have enough people to move the casualty safely and without further injury to hospital, you should leave the casualty where you found him.

If no doctor is coming:

Place loose pads between thighs, knees and ankles. Apply a figure-of-eight bandage to the feet and ankles. Place padding on the stretcher where the hollow of his neck and the hollow (small) of his back will be. The normal curves of the spine must be maintained. DO NOT use a pillow for his head.

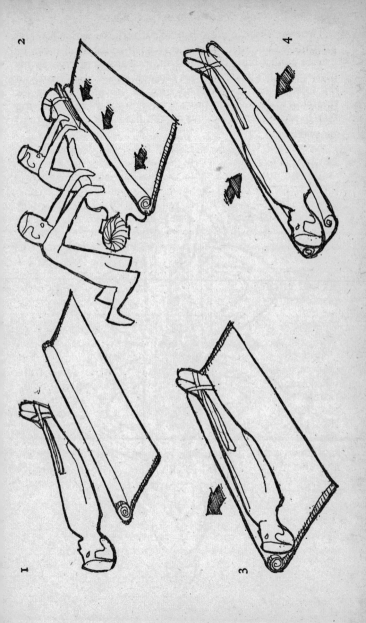

The easiest way to lift him on to a stretcher is with a blanket. First roll him on to his side so that a half-rolled blanket can be pushed under him. Next, roll the casualty gently on to his back again. The blanket edges can now be rolled up tightly to the sides of the casualty and used to provide purchase for several helpers. Lift the casualty straight up without allowing him to sag or twist. Pulling on the head and feet (traction)

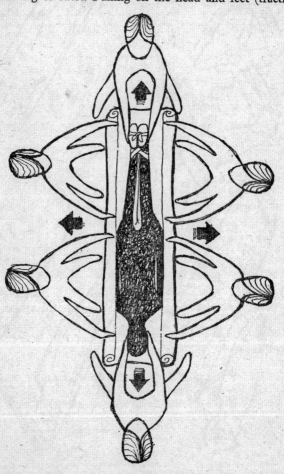

helps to keep the casualty straight. Now slide the stretcher in between the legs of one of the helpers at the head or feet and lower the casualty straight down on to the prepared stretcher.

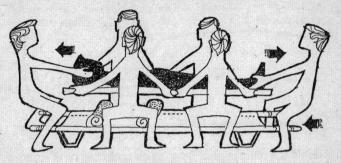

Lift without letting him sag

An improvised neck collar

If you think that the spine may be broken in the neck region, a stiff collar which can be made easily from a newspaper is very useful to prevent neck movement.

Fold the newspaper so that the width is about 4 inches – the same as the distance from the top of the casualty's breast bone to under the jaw.

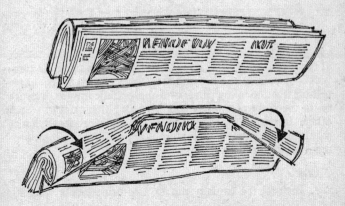

Place this collar around the neck, folding the newspaper over slightly to make the back edges narrower than the front. Overlap the ends around the neck.

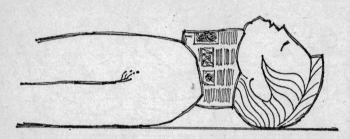

Hold the collar in place by using an encircling tie of string, a necktie or a bandage, tied over the top of the newspaper collar.

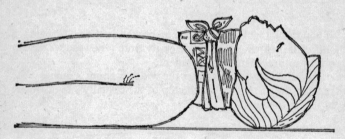

5. PELVIS

If the casualty has broken his thigh bone or his pelvis he complains of pain in the hip and sometimes the groin. A simple test for fracture of the pelvis is to apply gentle inward pressure on to the front of the hip bones pushing them towards each other. If the pelvis is fractured, the fracture site becomes painful immediately the pressure is applied. Any slight movement also indicates a fracture.

Treatment

1. Instruct the casualty not to pass urine before reaching

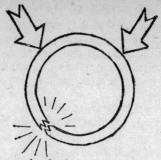

Compressing a ring leads to pain at the site of injury

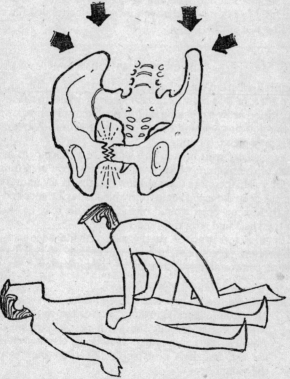

Pelvic ring-compression test for a fracture of the pelvis

hospital, even though he feels he must. Fracture of the pelvis often damages the urinary passage and if urine is passed, it will flow through the damaged area and spread into the tissues causing serious inflammation. If urine is passed, save a sample.

2. Lay him down in the most comfortable position – usually on his back.

3. Pad well between the knees and ankles.

4. Secure his knees together with a broad bandage.

5. Tie his feet and ankles together with a figure-of-eight bandage.

6. Send him to hospital on a stretcher without delay.

7. Serious internal bleeding sometimes occurs – so check frequently to make sure that you recognize concealed internal bleeding if it starts (p 53).

6. CHEST AND RIBS

Fractured ribs are caused most frequently by a fall on to a sharp edge, or by a blow from a car steering-wheel in a head-on car collision or by a crushing injury. A rib may also break when playing golf or coughing due to muscular action. A fragment of rib may pierce the lung.

The casualty with broken ribs will have a sharp pain in the region of the fracture which is increased on deep breathing or coughing. He therefore takes shallow breaths. If the underlying lung has been damaged some frothy blood may be coughed up.

If there is an open wound of the chest, air may be sucked into the chest and stop the lung working.

The muscles attached to the ribs provide adequate immobilization. Treatment, therefore, consists of making the casualty comfortable and treating any complications:

(i) Stop any serious bleeding.

(ii) If there is a wound of the chest which allows air to be sucked in (a 'sucking wound'), cover the wound *at once* with a sterile dressing. Seal it if possible with a large adhesive plaster dressing. If nothing else is available, use the casualty's own blood-stained clothing to plug the wound.

(iii) Send him to hospital quickly.

CONSCIOUS

(a) If he is conscious and not too distressed, send him in a sitting position.

(b) If this is uncomfortable, support him in a half-sitting position *on the injured side* or inclined towards the injured side. This leaves the uninjured lung free to work

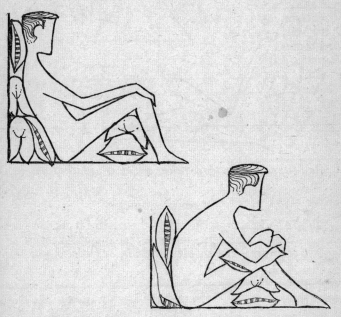

Sitting positions for conscious casualties with chest injuries. Incline to the injured side

normally, and allows any blood on the injured side to collect at the base of that lung.

(c) If both sides of the chest are injured, sit him up straight.

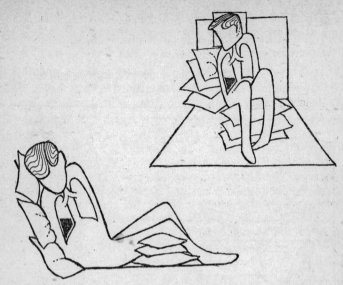

Half-sitting position for conscious casualties with chest injuries

UNCONSCIOUS

(*d*) If he is unconscious apply the treatment for any unconscious casualty – unconscious position, slight head-down tip – and lay him on the *injured* side.

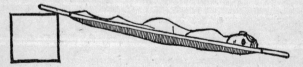

Lay the casualty on the injured *side*

DISLOCATIONS

A dislocation is present when a bone has been displaced at a joint from its normal position.

The *AIMS of FIRST-AID for DISLOCATIONS*
(*very similar to those for fractures*) *are to:*

Cover any wounds (dislocations may be closed or open).

Prevent any further injury by careful handling and immobilization.

Send the casualty to hospital.

THERE IS ONE EXTRA PRECAUTION – MAKE NO ATTEMPT TO REPLACE THE BONES INTO THEIR NORMAL POSITION. You will almost certainly make it worse.

A dislocation can only happen at a joint. When the ligaments and muscles which keep bones in position at a joint become torn, they allow the bones to become displaced from their normal position. A common site for this to happen is at the shoulder joint, where the arm bone may come right out of its socket in the shoulder blade.

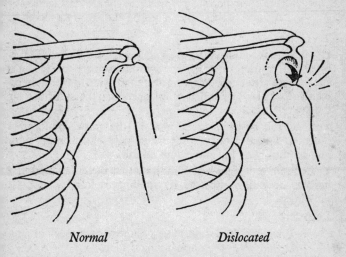

Normal   *Dislocated*

Dislocations often occur with or as a result of fractures. A fracture at the ankle may allow the ankle joint to dislocate.

In all cases of doubt, treat an injury at a joint as if it is a fraction or a dislocation or both.

Diagnosis

The diagnosis of joint injury is usually obvious.

(a) There is severe pain which may make the casualty feel sick.

(b) There is often swelling and bruising around the joint. This is caused by bleeding from the injured tissues.

(c) The displaced bone is often fixed in the position in which you find it by spasm of its attached muscles. The bone can only be moved with difficulty and then only with greatly increased pain.

(d) Other evidence is similar to that occurring with a fracture (which may, of course, also be present) such as tenderness and deformity (*see* page 103).

but (e) No grating of bone ends (crepitus) is present. This is because in a dislocation the bones which are displaced from their normal position usually are damaged very little and so there are no broken ends to grate together.

Treatment

1. Support the joint in the most comfortable position. This is often the position in which you find it. Support may mean a sling for an arm or securing the arm to the side of the body by bandages. Pillows or rolled-up blankets may be sufficient for the lower limbs.

2. Send the casualty to hospital in the most comfortable position. This is usually in the sitting position for upper limb injuries and lying for lower limb injuries.

3. Look for any signs which indicate that the circulation in a limb is becoming impaired by swelling, deformity or tight dressings.

Look for:

(i) Blue or white extremities (fingers and toes) or any change from the normal pink colour.

(ii) Loss of feeling below the injury. Test by asking the casualty if he can feel light touch in his fingertips and toes.

(iii) No pulse at the wrist or ankle.

If there is any doubt about circulation, loosen all tight dressings and straighten out the limb. Elbows are especially dangerous when bent. Tell the doctor immediately after you get the casualty to hospital about any troubles with circulation which you have observed.

Pneumatic inflatable splinting

This method of splinting limb fractures is easy to apply, can be applied over dressings, and is comfortable for the casualty. The splint, which is a double-layered tube of plastic, is zipped on to the limb and then inflated by mouth (not by pump as this may give too high a pressure). The splint then conforms to the shape of the limb and supports it. Being made of transparent material, the colour of the limb can be observed through the splint and any bleeding can be seen.

Pneumatic inflatable splints are only suitable for injuries which extend from just above the knee to the foot or from just above the elbow to the hand. For any injury much above the elbow or knee, these splints will not give suitable support.

The advantages of pneumatic inflatable splints are convenience and comfort. The disadvantages are their limited usefulness, their relatively high cost, and the fact that they can be punctured before (in which case they cannot be used) or while in use.

Summary of first-aid for FRACTURES

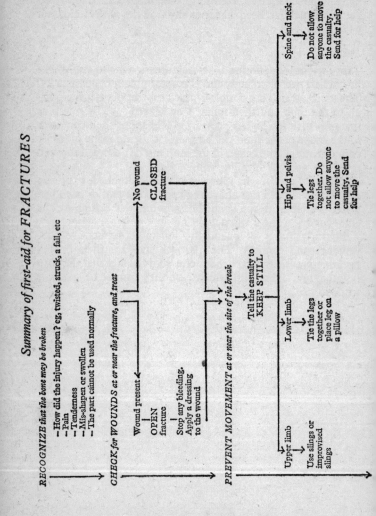

RECOGNIZE *that the bone may be broken*
— How did the injury happen? eg, twisted, struck, a fall, etc
— Pain
— Tenderness
— Mis-shapen or swollen
— The part cannot be used normally

CHECK *for WOUNDS at or near the fracture, and treat*

Wound present
OPEN fracture
Stop any bleeding. Apply a dressing to the wound

No wound
CLOSED fracture

PREVENT MOVEMENT *at or near the site of the break*

Tell the casualty to KEEP STILL

Upper limb
Use slings or improvised slings

Lower limb
Tie the legs together or place leg on a pillow

Hip and pelvis
Tie legs together. Do not allow anyone to move the casualty. Send for help

Spine and neck
Do not allow anyone to move the casualty. Send for help

Chapter 9

HEAD INJURIES

Many serious head injuries occur nowadays on the roads. Much can still be done to avert brain injury by motor-cyclists and scooter riders wearing 'skid lids', and by motorists using seat

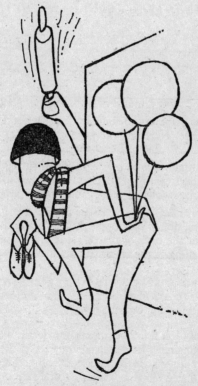

. . . in anticipation of possible injury !

belts. At work, hard hats perform a similar useful protection function. These articles must, however, be worn *before* the danger arises, in anticipation of possible injury.

If a head injury does occur, and there is any departure *whatsoever* from full normal alertness and responsiveness (full consciousness) for *however short a time*, it must be assumed that this is due to brain damage resulting from the injury. Many head injuries result in unconsciousness. An unconscious casualty may die within four minutes from *obstructed breathing* unless suitable first-aid is carried out.

The AIMS of FIRST-AID for HEAD INJURIES are to:

*Recognize obstructed breathing *at once* and treat it correctly.

*Apply the rules for the treatment of unconsciousness (*see* page 71).

Arrange for swift removal of the casualty to hospital.

Write down some notes which indicate the *level of consciousness* at the time. Note any *changes in the level of consciousness* together with the time of the change.

Watch continuously for any signs of obstructed breathing or unconsciousness coming on during the journey to hospital and take appropriate action if these conditions appear.

Obstructed breathing may come on *immediately* following unconsciousness, due to the tongue falling back and blocking the air passage at the back of the throat or *later* due to vomit or blood or frothing in the air passages.

OBSTRUCTED BREATHING IS PREVENTABLE BY FIRST-AID TREATMENT applied correctly and swiftly following injury.

As a result of careful investigations into deaths on the roads, it has been estimated that about one quarter of the people who become unconscious die from obstructed breathing – mainly as a result of inhaled blood or vomit. No other cause of death was

* These are life-saving measures if applied swiftly and correctly.

found: these people died because they were unconscious and, therefore, could not cough the obstructing matter out of their air passages. These lives can be saved by following the simple rules for the treatment of unconsciousness.

The treatment of obstructed breathing

1. Without moving the casualty, quickly remove any false teeth, or natural ones which have been knocked out. Wipe away any blood or vomit which may be obstructing the mouth or throat.

2. Gently bend the head back *fully* and support the lower jaw with the casualty's teeth clenched, as you would do to apply artificial respiration. This will allow the casualty to breathe *if he can*.

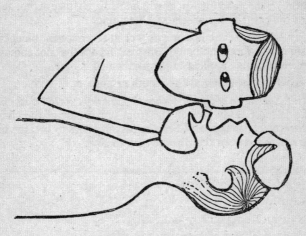

Listen for breathing

3. Watch and listen carefully (by placing your ear near his mouth and nose) for a few seconds to check whether the casualty can now breathe.

| IF HE CAN BREATHE treat as any unconscious casualty by turning the casualty into the *unconscious* position (keeping the head fully back) and if possible apply a slight head-down tip (*see* Chapter 4, page 71 for full details). | IF HE CANNOT BREATHE *apply artificial respiration* (*see* Chapter 3, page 41 for full details). |

Obstructed breathing can be recognized *by looking for*:

(i) *Noisy breathing.* It is a safe rule in first-aid to assume that *noisy breathing is obstructed breathing* until and unless shown otherwise.

The noise may be snoring or snorting or may be wheezy in type. Noisy breathing is a sign of airway obstruction, and on hearing it the good first-aider will immediately take action and treat the casualty for obstructed breathing.

(ii) *Blueness* of the lips or ears – or in severe cases, blueness of the whole face (and body). Blueness means that not enough oxygen is being supplied to the part which is blue.

(iii) *Frothing* either at the mouth or nose, or at both.

(iv) *Sucking in of the chest when the casualty tries to breathe in.* This is most easily seen in the front upper part of the chest below the collar bones. When the casualty tries to breathe in, the spaces between the ribs are seen to sink.

A note on normal breathing

A casualty who:

— is breathing quietly and easily;

— has pink lips and ears;

— has no froth around the nose or mouth;

is breathing normally and has no obstruction of the airway.

Attention should, therefore, be directed to any other conditions which are in need of treatment.

The reader may wonder why, in a chapter on head injuries,

the first section is spent on a discussion of obstructed breathing and the treatment of unconsciousness. This has been done in order to emphasize the importance which attaches to these conditions and to their correct treatment.

Here is an area where good first-aid, properly carried out, can indeed be life-saving. Failure to recognize and treat obstructed breathing in an unconscious casualty and to allow the airway to become obstructed by vomit or blood (by failing to follow the simple rules for treating unconsciousness) may cause a death which could have been avoided.

It should always be remembered that breathing which has once become obstructed requires careful and repeated checking to see that breathing remains normal and that the general condition of the casualty remains good.

In our discussion of head injuries we can now, having dealt with the first 'B' – 'breathing' – go on to discuss the second 'B' – 'brain damage'.

Brain damage can be caused in three main ways.

(i) *By a penetrating injury or by a depressed fracture of the skull*

These injuries may be caused by a sharp or pointed object such as a car handle or mascot, or the sharp edge of some piece of metal, concrete or stone. The object may penetrate the skull and injure the brain, or cause a depressed fracture of the skull. The fragments of depressed bone will either penetrate or press on to the brain, thus causing damage. Such injuries usually cause brain damage in a small area of the brain. As a result of this type of injury, there may be bleeding inside the skull [*see* (ii) below].

(ii) *By bleeding inside the skull*

This bleeding may give rise to a clot or collection of blood inside the skull. The skull can be regarded as a hard bony box with a limited space inside it which is occupied by the brain. If the brain, which is soft, is compressed by blood, serious damage may ensue.

Bleeding may arise due to a wound from a sharp object as in (i) above, or the bleeding may occur following an injury by a blunt object – for example the head may strike the road. Bleeding in this case is due to tearing of a blood vessel inside the skull. Such injuries may or may not be accompanied by immediate unconsciousness or by a fracture of the skull.

(iii) *By an injury which results in a sudden violent movement of the head or, when the head is moving, results in a sudden stopping of movement.*

Examples of these would be a blow on the point of the jaw and a crash into a brick wall at twenty miles an hour. In these cases, the brain is not directly injured, nothing presses on or penetrates into the brain. The injury is the result of indirect violence.

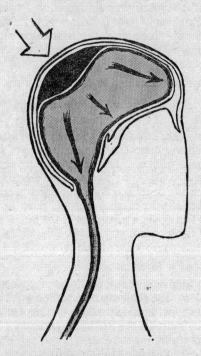

Blood may compress the brain

A useful way of thinking about how this damage arises is to liken the brain to a soft jelly inside a mould. Shaking of the mould or sudden stopping of movement – for example by throwing the mould against a wall – will result in damage to the jelly. This damage will be mainly on the outside of the jelly where it meets the mould, at, and also opposite to, the point of impact. However, damage will also occur throughout the jelly in most cases. The sequence of events which follows this type of brain injury is immediate unconsciousness followed by recovery in favourable cases. The name for this kind of injury is *concussion* – more commonly known as a 'knock-out'.

Brain damage can, therefore, be recognized:

– *By the presence of a penetrating wound or a depressed fracture*

– *By any departure whatever from full normal alertness for however short a time or however slight an amount.*

It is usual to describe varying degrees of unconsciousness. For example, the casualty may be completely unconscious and incapable of being roused. On the other hand he may be in a dreamy and confused state, yet able to answer questions more or less reasonably. If we think of full normal alertness (normal consciousness) as WHITE, and unrousable unconsciousness (deep unconsciousness) as BLACK, we can immediately recognize that every shade of GREY may exist in between. There is, therefore, no reason to name or to describe any particular stages as if they were fixed points. What matters in any head injury, with or without loss of consciousness, is to find:

THE LEVEL OF CONSCIOUSNESS, and to note
ANY CHANGE IN THE LEVEL.

The level of consciousness can be simply described in everyday language. For example, 'fully alert', 'completely normal in speech and manner', or 'rather confused, responds to questions slowly and with difficulty, appears to want to go off to sleep', or 'after a fit which appeared to affect the right arm and leg, he lapsed into deep unconsciousness and could not be roused to speech or movement, even when pinched'.

Fully conscious	White
Slightly dreamy and confused	Very light grey
Mildly unconscious but can be roused to speech	Light grey
Unconscious, will move on stimulation	Mid grey
Unconscious, cannot be roused to speech or movement	Dark grey
Deeply unconscious, shallow breathing	Very dark grey
Deeply unconscious, not breathing, large pupils	Black

Having described the level of consciousness at any point in time, the next important thing is to watch for any change in the level of consciousness (or general condition) of the casualty. If there is, the direction of the change should be carefully noted, ie, whether the degree of unconsciousness is becoming deeper or lighter.

Remember:

All casualties who have any loss of consciousness for however short a time should be seen by a doctor. Any casualty who, following a head injury, appears to be becoming more unconscious should be taken *without delay* to hospital, in the unconscious position with a slight head-down tip.

Chapter 10

POISONING

Poisons are substances which can harm the body. Accidental poisoning by mouth is avoidable and, in the majority of cases, can easily be prevented. It is one of the more common causes of death in young children. Take action now to PREVENT poisoning:

(*a*) Store poisons in properly labelled containers well out of reach of children in a *locked* cupboard or drawer.

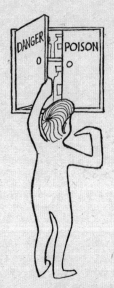

Store poisons well out of reach of children

(*b*) Most tablets, pills and capsules are brightly coloured and attractive to children. LOCK THEM AWAY.

(c) DO NOT take drinks or medicines in the dark. First look at the label in a good light.

(d) DO NOT keep medicines, lotions and pills for a long time. Throw old medicines away by emptying them down the lavatory, and so make sure that they are not available to children.

(e) Household cleaners, paraffin, etc. should be stored in such a way that children (especially the under fours) *cannot* drink them.

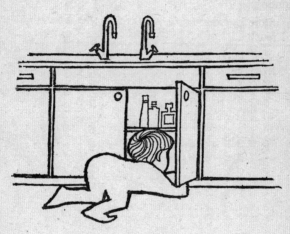

Lock away household cleaners

Proper first-aid started promptly can often do more to ensure recovery than skilled medical treatment given after the poison has begun to take effect.

The table following gives the first-aid treatment for poisoning by mouth.

Casualties who become unconscious following poisoning by mouth may sometimes have fits (convulsions). The treatment for fits is given on page 75.

FIRST-AID FOR POISONING BY MOUTH

I. ACT QUICKLY

2. (i) IF UNCONSCIOUS

Treat as any unconscious casualty (*see* Chapter 5 for full details). Unconscious position with a slight head-down tip, and send quickly to hospital, together with any clues as to what the poison may be, such as tablets, empty bottles or vomited material, etc

(ii) IF CONSCIOUS

WHAT is the POISON?

if the poison causes BURNING OF THE LIPS, MOUTH or TONGUE or if the poison is a PETROLEUM PRODUCT

→ Send quickly to hospital

DO NOT make the casualty VOMIT

→ Give ice-cream or one tablespoon of vegetable oil (olive oil, cooking oil). Petroleum products are not dangerous unless they get into the lungs because of vomiting – so try not to do anything which may make the casualty vomit. Now send to hospital

For ALL OTHER POISONS

Except as Above

MAKE the casualty **VOMIT** by giving

- 15 ml of ipecac syrup*

OR

- two tablespoonsful of salt in a glass of warm water†

OR

- two teaspoonsful of mustard in a glass of warm water†

OR

- put a finger down his throat (his finger or yours) to depress the tongue and touch the back of the throat

DILUTE any remaining poison, then

Give two or three glasses of water or other bland fluid such as milk, lemonade, etc

SEND QUICKLY TO HOSPITAL

ALWAYS SEND CLUES TO HOSPITAL with the casualty.

Send empty bottles, tablets, vomited material, berries or anything else which you think may help the doctors in hospital to identify the poison and the dose

 See note on page 148.

† *It is **dangerous** to give more than the recommended dose.*

The use of ipecac syrup to make children vomit

If a child should be made to vomit after taking a poison (*see* pages 146–7 for details of which poisons to treat in this way), 15 ml of ipecac syrup USP* is probably the best thing to use as an emetic.

As a means of removing poison from the stomachs of young children ipecac syrup is suitable for home use and is much *faster* acting than sending a child to hospital for a stomach wash-out; it is also more *effective* than a stomach wash-out.

After giving 15 ml of ipecac syrup, the child should be given a drink of water and should be kept moving until he vomits; movement aids the onset of vomiting. After vomiting, proceed as instructed on pages 146–7.

* Ipecac syrup USP is –

powdered ipecac	7 grammes
glycerine	10 ml
syrup	100 ml

Other preparations of ipecac should NOT be used to induce vomiting. The SYRUP only should be used.

Chapter 11

WET-COLD CHILLING and IMMERSION CHILLING

Heat loss from the body, with lowering of body temperature, is the reason for illness or death following exposure to wet-cold conditions or due to immersion in cold water.

Death from wet-cold chilling (exposure) in hilly or mountainous country is sufficiently frequent to warrant a mention. Practically all cases are due to inadequate equipment and lack of appreciation that exposure to wet-cold can kill even well-trained, uninjured adults. Let no walker forget that even in summer, arctic conditions may very quickly arise in hilly country, and find the hiker ill-prepared for a night out.

Heat loss from the body is the reason for wet-cold chilling illness or death. Severe chilling can result in death within two hours.

Prevention

(i) *Equipment*

Waterproof clothing and over-garments would prevent most wet-cold chilling casualties. Plasticized nylon is cheap, and trousers, anoraks, mackintoshes and capes made in this material are easily obtainable. Such waterproof clothing is light in weight, small in bulk, and can be easily packed and carried. It is, of course, less serviceable for regular wear than heavier waterproof garments, but is well suited for occasional use.

Condensation occurs inside plasticized nylon garments in cold weather. They should therefore be as loose as possible to assist ventilation. It seems likely that if they are worn over ordinary windproof garments the latter would be sufficiently water-resistant to prevent the moisture penetrating inwards.

The effects of head and face covering should never be forgotten. About 20 per cent of the heat from the body can be lost in this way, while the rest of the body is clothed. Fur and leather helmets, sou'westers and balaclavas all have an important role in the prevention of heat loss from these areas.

Reserve clothing – for example, an extra pair of thick socks, ski socks, a warm sweater, an extra pair of trousers and a pair of gloves – should be carried in the rucksack *in a waterproof plastic bag* in order to keep the clothing bone-dry. This reserve clothing will only be of use if it can be kept dry before use and when worn. Extra trousers as well as sweaters should always be included.

A large, lightweight, waterproof cape in which you can bivouac, and a large wound-dressing (No 15, BPC) are useful items.

A *torch* and a *whistle* should also be carried so as to be able to attract attention in case of collapse, injury or other trouble.

Brightly coloured clothing should be chosen and worn. Experience has shown that dull colours merge into the surroundings, and if rescue becomes necessary casualties are harder to find.

The commonest deficiencies of the usually accepted clothing are:

(a) lack of protection against wetting;

(b) insufficient insulation and resistance to wind penetration over the legs.

Emergency rations should always be carried, eg, chocolate, glucose, or other compressed rations of high calorie content.

A polythene bag (7 feet by 4 feet, 500 gauge), which can be used as a windproof, waterproof covering for any casualty, should be included in the equipment of any group.

(ii) *Shelter*

If the weather worsens or any member of a party shows any likelihood of becoming wet or tired, shelter should be sought AT ONCE. It is foolish to wait until exhaustion and collapse occur before seeking shelter.

Camping may be a means of providing shelter, provided that the members of the party have sufficient experience and adequate equipment to remain warm and dry in camp.

When a person shows any early signs of wet–cold chilling

(see below) the surest way of preventing disaster is to camp at once.

(iii) *Leadership*

No party, particularly of young people, should venture out in wild, open, or mountainous country without adequately trained and experienced leaders or guides. *Never go alone.*

(iv) *Obtain a weather forecast before setting out*

The weather centre can be contacted by telephone. Before setting out, it is wise to obtain a *detailed* and *up-to-date* forecast from the nearest weather centre – see the telephone directory for details.

(v) *Fitness*

Reasonable physical fitness is essential. Neglect of this obvious factor leads to needless tragedies.

(vi) *Inform others of the intended route*

Always inform some responsible person of the intended route and the expected time of arrival at the destination. Such information is vital should rescue become necessary. Any would-be rescuer must make sure that he does not himself become a casualty through being inadequately trained, prepared, or equipped.

(vii) *Load carrying*

The maximum weight that anyone should carry is 40 lbs (18 kg) *or* one-third of his own weight, whichever is the lesser figure.

How to recognize wet–cold chilling in the early stages

— Be aware that wet–cold chilling may occur.

— Abnormal behaviour is often an early indication; the casualty may become uncooperative, dreamy and slow in his responses, or apathetic. Any departure from normal behaviour should be viewed with suspicion.

— Weakness, slowing, excessive tiredness, stumbling and repeated falling appear, probably in that order.

In the late stages

— Collapse, stupor and unconsciousness occur, and may go on to death.

— Cramp, loss of sensation in the legs, loss of movement and fits also occur in some cases.

The AIMS of FIRST-AID for WET-COLD CHILLING are to provide:

— insulation

— rest, and

— shelter.

Insulation will conserve body heat and allow natural heat production to raise body temperature. *Rest* will allow natural heat production, which may be slowed or stopped by exhaustion, to begin again. *Shelter* will prevent worsening and will assist in the other two aims of providing rest and insulation.

Cooling by evaporation must be avoided

Even small amounts of air movement will cause rapid evaporation and thus cooling of the casualty. A gale may refrigerate him. Provided that the casualty is wrapped in an outer windproof, impermeable layer such as a polythene sack, plus plenty of insulation such as blankets or coats, it does not matter how wet the clothes and skin are. When cooling by evaporation is stopped by a windproof, impermeable layer, the natural heat production of the body should be enough to cause a rise in body temperature.

First-aid for wet–cold chilling

This will usually have to be carried out in adverse physical conditions such as on a moor or mountainside. The casualty or casualties will often be exhausted as well as chilled.

If one or a number of any party are thought to be suffering

from wet–cold chilling, immediate action should be taken as follows:

— Stop, and rest the casualty. Make a camp and try to shelter him (or them) from the wind and weather. Keep the casualty lying down. It is much better to shelter *immediately* and make efforts to deal with the condition than to transport the person untreated to a hospital or other distant place of shelter. Because the illness is caused by chilling, by exhaustion and by loss of body heat, the sooner these can be reversed, the better are the chances of a favourable outcome.

— Insulate the casualty immediately, where he is, by getting him into a sleeping-bag or rolled in blankets. Do not disturb his clothing.

— Complete the casualty's insulating cocoon by adding a windproof layer (a large polythene bag, 7 feet by 4 feet, 500 gauge) on the outside. Place the casualty – in the sleeping-bag or wrapped in blankets – inside the poly-thene bag. Remember also to cover his head and forehead with a helmet or cap and to insulate his neck with a scarf – much heat can be lost if this is not done.

— Insulate well *under* the casualty. Much heat will be lost into the ground if this is not done.

— If the casualty is removed from rain and wind to shelter, apply additional outer layers of insulation. *Do not* remove the wet clothes and the insulating cocoon until the casualty has recovered and is responding normally.

— Give warm drinks and sugary foods if the casualty is conscious and these can be provided.

— If the casualty is recovering – and most casualties will recover if insulated, rested and sheltered – he will not come to further harm if he is kept where he is. Be pre-pared for a long wait until proper help arrives.

— If stretcher transport has to be used, try to maintain a slight head-down tip.

— An ambulance, or other suitable vehicle in which the casualty can be transported lying down, should be brought as near to the casualty as possible to avoid the disadvantage of a long stretcher journey.

Chapter 12

HOW TO APPROACH AND PLAN FOR AN INCIDENT

1. *How long will it take before the casualty is safely in hospital?*

In approaching any incident, it is helpful to have an idea of *how long* it will take to get any casualties to skilled medical treatment in hospital. This basic fact may affect to some extent *what* is to be done and *how* it is to be done. For example, a casualty who has a broken ankle which occurs in a busy street a few hundred yards from a large hospital should, normally, arrive there after a smooth journey with the minimum of delay. To transport the same casualty from the middle of a wild and lonely stretch of hill country would, of necessity, entail a longer and much rougher journey.

2. *What help is immediately available?*

All available resources must be utilized. To do this, the first-aider should ask himself:

   (i) how many people, including children, are available and can help?

  (ii) what kind of people are they? Are they trained first-aiders, or calm sensible adults, or excitable people, or young adults who, given a clear message, can deliver it quickly?

 (iii) is there any transport available, such as a car or a lorry, or any other equipment which may be useful?

 (iv) how can I best make use of the available resources?

3. *How many casualties?*

The next problem will be to assess the total situation – is there one casualty or many? Are the casualties in a situation of danger – or can they remain where they are until suitable first-aid treatment has been carried out? If there are multiple casualties, the first thing to be done is to make sure that the police or ambulance authorities are alerted in order that they can summon adequate help. A brief description of the incident together with an assessment of the number of casualties is all that will be required. The police and ambulance authorities will then do the rest.

Some forms of incident result in a scattering of casualties – for example high-speed car crashes. It is important that casualties are sought for in the surrounding area – particularly at night. Those most in need of help will probably be the ones who have been flung out of the car. Those who remain in the car, particularly if wearing seat belts, will:

(i) be found;
(ii) tend to be less seriously injured than any passengers from the same vehicle who are thrown out, or passengers from other vehicles who fall out.

The important point to remember is *always look for other casualties, particularly at night*.

4. *Onerous decisions*

The well trained first-aider in approaching any incident will NOT spend a long time attending to the first casualty he finds *unless* he has ascertained that this is the only casualty. He will:

(i) assess the total situation;
(ii) assess the help which is immediately available;
(iii) assess the total number of casualties, after searching for stragglers or arranging for a search to be made;
(iv) make a decision about the need to summon help, and arrange for a clear message to be passed to the police and ambulance authorities;
(v) then seek out the casualties who are likely to benefit most by first-aid at this time.

Who are these likely to be? In any incident with multiple casualties there may be a wide range of casualties, from those who are dead or dying to those who are badly shaken and have relatively minor injuries. None of these groups fall into the category of casualties who are likely to benefit most by first-aid treatment. The obviously dying should be left. This sounds inhuman; but, in the context of limited help in a disaster situation, it is the only reasonable course to follow. Those who can be saved must have prior attention.

Similarly, the lightly injured should be left: their lives are not in danger and they do not need immediate assistance. Come back to them, after you have dealt with the casualties whose lives you may be able to save and after seeking out the casualties who must be taken to hospital first when help arrives.

Correct and quick sorting out of casualties in the early stages can save lives.

What conditions can best be helped by first-aid at this stage?

Unconsciousness and obstructed breathing

Any casualty who is *unconscious* (and breathing) should be placed in the unconscious position with a head-down tip if possible, following the rules for the treatment of unconsciousness.

Bleeding

Any casualties who are *bleeding* or who have *large wounds* should have dressings firmly applied to stop bleeding, following the rules for wounds and bleeding. Unskilled assistance could, for example, arrange to keep limbs elevated if this was required.

Multiple injuries

Other injuries which are judged to be severe or multiple should then be treated.

All casualties in the above categories should be listed (mentally or on paper – again the unskilled assistant could help) and when medical help or ambulances arrive, the correct order of priorities for sending the casualties to hospital should be easy to work out.

5. Improvisation and leadership

It is not possible in a brief description such as we have attempted above to give more than an outline of principles and priorities. However, with an understanding of principles and priorities, together with the skilled first-aid, AND good improvisation and leadership, much can be accomplished.

In emergency situations of any kind, people are always ready to help but they may not know what to do. If you can see clearly what should be done, do not hesitate to ask or tell others what to do. People will follow a lead, if they understand that the leader knows more than they do. Never try to do everything yourself. Use every bit of help you can get. If people do not offer to help, and you think that they could, do not hesitate to ask them. As a general rule they will respond willingly, but you must tell them *clearly* what you want them to do.

The comments which have been made above refer to the situation which is most common in first-aid – when no doctor is present. However, if a doctor is present or if someone else has more skill and experience than you, accept orders and instructions from them.

ROAD CRASHES

Because road crashes are, unfortunately, so common, we include here a few brief suggestions about how to tackle the problems which arise from such incidents. Much of the material has already appeared in other parts of the book – but most of the lessons are worth repetition.

The AIMS of RESCUERS dealing with a ROAD CRASH are to:

Protect the scene of the incident;
Alert the rescue services;
Give first-aid.

Protect the scene of the incident

This must be given *top priority* in order to prevent further casualties caused by on-coming vehicles either running over lightly injured people who are lying in the road, or running into rescuers. Some of the things which can be done are:

— Send someone to park a car and to signal to traffic to slow down in one or both directions from the incident.

— Place red warning triangles on the road.

— Switch off engines and ignition of all vehicles to prevent fire.

— Enforce no smoking or striking of matches to prevent fire. If you see or smell petrol appoint a fire warden to watch for fire and to enforce no smoking.

— Use the lights of undamaged vehicles to illuminate the crash scene.

— At night wear something white or fluorescent if possible. Stick a newspaper under a collar or belt at night to produce a white conspicuous patch against dark clothing.

Alert the rescue services

This may be done by people who cannot do first-aid while those trained in first-aid attend to the casualties.

Dial 999 and give a clear message to include:

— How many *badly* injured and *lightly* injured casualties.

— Whether extrication of trapped casualties may be required.

— Where *exactly* the crash is, or the *exact* location of the telephone from which you are speaking – all public telephone boxes have this information displayed, and motorway telephones are numbered.

— What services you think may be required, for example, three ambulances and a crane to lift a car.

Give first-aid

Give the life-saving first-aid for

— not breathing
— bleeding, and
— unconsciousness.

Many people die needlessly from obstructed breathing as a result of a short period of unconsciousness following road crashes. If there are many casualties do a quick check on each one and carry out life-saving first-aid *before* doing first-aid for other conditions and before looking in detail for other injuries. If those priorities are not observed, lives may be lost needlessly.

Resist the inclination of untrained people to drag casualties out of vehicles. The only indication for immediate removal, regardless of injuries, is that the vehicle is on fire. Most fires occur very shortly after the crash. If there is no fire and the precautions outlined previously for protecting the scene of the incident are followed, it is very unlikely that there will be a fire. Casualties should therefore be left in the vehicles until they can be removed skilfully, slowly and with care in case they have neck, spinal or other serious injuries. They will also be protected from the weather if left inside – and this may be important. One blanket can be used to conserve body heat.

Talk quietly, calmly and reassuringly to casualties until the ambulance arrives. Avoid gruesome details of what has happened to other people.

Never permit panic handling of any casualty, however well-meaning is the intention of the untrained people who try to do this.

If a casualty is on the ground, always have a thick coat or blanket *under* him. If there is only one coat or blanket, use this *under* the casualty; more body heat can be conserved in this way than by using the coat or blanket to cover the casualty.

At night, always search the area of a crash *and around it* for people who have been thrown out of vehicles. Try to account for each occupant of every vehicle; those who have been thrown out may be the ones most in need of help.

Experience of many road crashes shows that

— The short time spent in getting priorities properly evaluated can save lives.
— More deliberation and less panic handling would be beneficial.

Chapter 13

HOME TREATMENT

This chapter deals with minor injuries or illnesses where the aim of treatment will be to do everything necessary *without* passing the casualty on to hospital or to a doctor. The treatment, if all goes well, will be *final* – not *first* (aid).

WOUNDS

(i) *Self-help* – follows the same lines as home treatment.
(ii) *Home treatment*

Only minor wounds should be treated, such as small cuts, lacerations or 'gravel rash'. The amount of surface damage is not necessarily a good guide to the severity of the wound. Stab and puncture wounds can cause deep injuries of a serious nature. They are also the means by which infection can be conveyed to the inside of the body. The *skin* wound may be minor in such cases, but these injuries should always be regarded seriously, especially those in the head and neck, around joints and near body cavities such as the chest or abdomen, and in the hand. *As a general rule, if you think that the depth of penetration may be beyond the thickness of the skin which covers the part* (and you can tell the skin depth by picking it up and feeling the thickness between your fingers) *you should apply first-aid, and take the casualty to be seen by a doctor.*

The aims of *home treatment* of wounds are very similar to the aims of *first-aid* treatment of wounds (*see* page 59).

The AIMS of HOME TREATMENT for WOUNDS are to:

Stop bleeding.

Carry out adequate wound cleaning – *both* the wound *and* the surrounding skin.

Apply a suitable dressing. This should be allowed to remain in place until healing has occurred.

1. *How to stop bleeding* is dealt with on page 57.

2. *Wound cleaning*

Adequate wound cleaning is by far the most important step in securing sound wound healing. It is often the least well carried out step by those who are not medically trained.

The principles of adequate wound cleaning are:

   (i) Do not introduce infection into the wound.

  (ii) Remove any obvious dirt, foreign material and dead tissues from the wound (scissors may be required to trim off dead skin for example).

 (iii) Clean the surrounding skin, keeping the wound covered.

 (iv) Clean the wound thoroughly.

(i) *Do not introduce infection into the wound* while cleaning it. In practice, under home conditions, this means that no attempt should be made to clean up any wound until your hands have been thoroughly washed. It is best then to shake the hands well and dry them lightly on the inside of a clean towel. If possible the hands should not touch the wound. Care should also be taken not to cough or sneeze while treatment is being carried out.

Ideally all equipment and dressings should be sterile, and the wound cleaning and dressing should be applied by a 'no-touch' technique. At home, dressings can be sterile. The method of cleaning should aim to minimize contact of the operator's skin with the wound, cleansers and dressings. All equipment used should be as clean as possible.

(ii) *Wipe away any obvious dirt and remove any loose pieces of foreign material such as wood or metal which are in the wound.* Remove any dead skin (or other dead tissue) by trimming off with scissors. These things should be done before proceeding to clean the surrounding skin or the wound.

(iii) *Clean the surrounding skin.* Begin by covering the wound. Then start to clean an area about two inches away from the wound. Use plenty of swabs. Discard at once any swab which becomes dirty, or is moistened with blood or sticky fluid from the wound. Wipe the dirt outwards and away from the wound. Then clean more closely to the wound edges until you have to

uncover the wound in order to clean the skin edges of the
wound. Do not allow the cleaning fluid to run from the skin
into or on to the wound as infection might be conveyed into it.
We recommend a cetrimide-containing detergent cleaner such
as 'Savlon' (*see* Appendix 1 for the kit required for home
treatment).

It is as important to clean the surrounding skin thoroughly
as it is to clean the wound, because infection can reach the

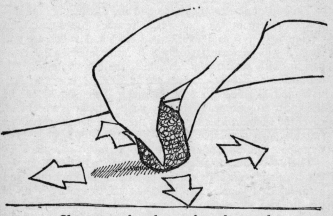

Clean outwards and away from the wound

wound from the surrounding skin. It may also be wise, if the
skin is hairy, to shave the hairs for a distance of *at least* one
inch from the wound margins.

(iv) *Clean the wound thoroughly*

Self-help is often the best way to accomplish thorough wound
cleaning, provided that the end result is adequately supervised
and no skimping of the cleaning-up process is accepted.

If possible, casualties should be given a supply of *running*
water. If this is not available, several basinsful (which should
be changed as the cleaning proceeds) and cleaning materials
(diluted 'Savlon' is best, but soap and water will do very well)
should be provided. Each casualty should be instructed to

scrub till clean and will usually make a very good job of the cleaning, provided that he is allowed to take his time and is not hurried. He must, however, be carefully supervised and kept up to the mark in terms of the final result! In these circumstances the casualty can judge the amount of pain which he is willing to suffer against the inconvenience of being kept at the job of cleaning until the desired result is forthcoming. Self-help here is the best method if it can be used. It is particularly suitable for children.

Time spent on cleaning the wound and the surrounding skin is time well spent. Wounds which are free of dead tissue and foreign matter (dirt, metal, wood, etc) and which are well cleaned will heal satisfactorily and resist infection by comparison with similar wounds which are not treated in this manner.

Wound cleaning must be thorough. Pain should *not* be allowed to stop proper efforts at cleaning. If pain is a problem, cover the wound with a temporary dressing, give the casualty a suitable dose of soluble aspirin (*see* Appendix 1, page 175), wait about ten minutes and then start again.

There is nothing to be gained and much to be lost by applying dressings, antiseptic creams or lotions on top of dirty and germ-infected wounds. The effect of such 'treatment' is to seal the dirt and germs into the wound. Part of nature's defence mechanism is to shed any dead tissue and pus (which includes germs) to the surface of a wound. Nothing should therefore be done to interfere with this mechanism, and all possible steps should be taken to aid it.

For this and other reasons we believe that

ADEQUATE WOUND CLEANING IS THE MOST IMPORTANT STEP IN SECURING GOOD HEALING OF ANY WOUND.

Attention is called to the dressings which are recommended; they are STERILE, *not* antiseptic. These dressings allow natural healing to occur, provided that the previous steps have been properly carried out. The dressings carry almost no risk of allergy or reaction and are not painful or uncomfortable when applied. To make sure that antiseptics, ointments, lotions, iodine, germicides and so on are *not* available as a substitute for proper wound cleaning, we would suggest that they be consigned to your dustbin or poured down the lavatory!

Cotton-wool should *not* be used in contact with any wound or burn as it leaves behind stray fragments which have to be picked out of the wound or burn, but cannot be completely removed. These stray fragments act as foreign bodies and cause delayed healing. Cotton-wool fragments also carry and spread infection.

3. *Dress the wound.* Dressings should be put on, and, ideally, should remain in place until the wound is healed. This statement pre-supposes some knowledge about how to fix dressings in place and about wound-healing times. Most minor wounds should be healed or well on the way to healing by seven days.

Dressings can be held in place by roller bandages – conforming bandages are best – or crêpe bandages, by sticking plaster or by both sticking plaster and bandages. Occasionally, finger-stalls and other such devices may be helpful. Dressings should always be sterile (you should buy them like this). There are two main kinds of dressing:

(*a*) Dry (surgical gauze swab).
(*b*) Non-adhesive, (eg, vaseline net or other non-adhesive dressings – *see* page 175).

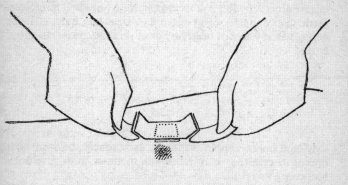

No-touch application of a sticky patch

The purpose of a dry dressing is to allow a dry seal to form on the surface of a wound. Dry dressings are the treatment of choice for *any* wound or burn where there is not an area of damaged skin surface which would stick to the dressing, making the removal of the dressing an unpleasant procedure. For the latter sort of wound a non-adhesive dressing is best.

Kind of wound	*Which dressing to use*
'clean cuts' by sharp instruments	dry
small surface burns	dry or non-adhesive
'gravel rash'	non-adhesive
irregular wounds, leaving some raw areas	non-adhesive

BURNS AND SCALDS
SELF-HELP

Shallow burns of small areas are the only types of burns or scalds which should be treated at home.

Burns should, after cooling the burn with water (*see* page 90), be treated like wounds by adequate cleaning. Clean the surrounding skin first, and then clean the burned skin. The choice of dry or non-adhesive dressing will be determined by the extent of raw areas left. Remember that skin loss needs skin replacement in hospital – so do not try to treat any burn at home which has any area of blistering or of skin *loss* greater than this circle.

Minor burns of the eyelids or face should be seen by a doctor in case they may cause loss of function or produce a bad cosmetic result.

Small burns are often very painful, so cover the burn with a temporary dry dressing and then give the casualty some pain reliever before you start proper treatment by cleaning and so on. Soluble aspirin is probably the cheapest, safest and best general-use pain reliever. The dosage is given in Appendix 1, paragraph 4, page 175.

SUNBURN

Probably the best application for minor sunburn (when the skin is red but not blistering) is calamine cream. This should be applied to the affected areas. Sunburn with blistering in any but small areas should be seen by a doctor.

BRUISES

A bruise is caused by bleeding into the tissues. Home treatment can only hope to minimize the effects – once the blow has been delivered there are bound to be consequences!

Ice packs, cold cloths (wrung out in cold water) and elevation of limbs together with a crêpe bandage applied from *below* the swelling to beyond and above it will all help. Rest also helps, particularly in the early stages, as this allows blood to clot and thus stops the bleeding (*see* page 57). Once a large, tense, painful swelling has developed the problem may require more than home treatment.

FOREIGN BODIES

Foreign bodies are things that should not be in the body (*see* page 61). They include wood splinters in the fingers, beads up the nose, grit in the eye, swallowed toys or buttons, and so on.

1. *Foreign bodies in wounds* should be removed if they are loose. *If stuck, they should be left* and first-aid treatment given (*see* page 61). Small splinters under the nail or skin should be removed by tweezers. Remember that these wounds can often be deep and that infection may be driven into the body. If the foreign body is much more than skin-deep, it is wise to have such wounds seen by a doctor. When you have removed the foreign body, clean the surrounding skin and the wound, and apply a dressing (*see* page 162).

2. Foreign body in the eye

(i) Self-help

Blink the eye rapidly once or twice. This may, by movement and as a result of the increased tear-flow which occurs due to eye irritation, allow the foreign body to be dislodged. If not, do not rub the eye – you will only make it worse. Next, gently pull the edge of the upper lid over the lower lid (grasp the upper eyelashes) and release. This may remove the foreign body. If you fail to remove the foreign body in this way, then put an eye pad over the eye and seek help.

(ii) Minor Treatment

Seat the casualty facing a good light. Have ready the corner of a clean handkerchief or a *moistened* cotton-wool-tipped applicator. Stand behind the casualty and ask the casualty to put his head back till his head leans against you. Search systematically for the foreign body.

Instructions to the Casualty	*Where to search*
1. Look up.	Under the lower lid.
2. Look to the right.	The left corner.
3. Look to the left.	The right corner.
4. Look down.	Pull the upper lid gently back until the lashes can be held against the bony ridge of the top of the eye socket. Look at the central and upper part of the eyeball and under the upper lid.
5. Look at my nose.	Look at the central part of the eyeball, particularly at the clear window part (the cornea).

Any foreign body which is seen should be gently wiped off with one wipe. If it does not come off or move with one wipe, then it is probably stuck to the eye. No attempt should be made to remove foreign bodies which are stuck to the eye. Cover the eye with a pad and bandage and send the casualty to hospital.

(*Chemical splashes* in the eye are dealt with on page 96).

3. *Foreign bodies in the nose and ear*

These usually occur in children. Make no attempt to remove the foreign body. Take the child to hospital. There is usually no immediate danger with beads and similar objects.

Do not pour water or oil into ears in an attempt to dislodge a foreign body. If the child persists in poking inside his ear, apply a pad and bandage.

4. *Inhaled foreign bodies*

These usually result in violent coughing. Place the casualty face down over the edge of a bed or table with the head down to allow the object to be expelled. If the foreign body remains inside or cannot be found, take the casualty to hospital at once.

If an object similar to the inhaled one can easily be found, take this to hospital with the casualty. It may make the work of the surgeon swifter and more effective. Remember, too, that if dentures are broken, or if natural teeth are chipped or missing, these objects may have been inhaled. Always seek medical advice *at once* and tell the doctor your suspicions.

5. *Swallowed foreign body* ('in the stomach')

This usually occurs in children. If there is any sign of choking, up-end the child and give a suitable tap on the back between the shoulder blades. This should dislodge the foreign body (often a sweet).

The danger of any swallowed object which does not cause choking and has gone right down, will depend on whether it is sharp-edged and pointed (such as an open safety-pin) – in which case it will be dangerous – or whether it is smooth and rounded (such as a marble) in which case it will not.

If the object is sharp, pointed, or jagged, medical aid should be sought at once. GIVE NOTHING BY MOUTH.

With smooth, round objects, a good working rule is that if the foreign body is small enough to be swallowed, then it will probably go right through. In the case of children under two years old, it is best to see a doctor as at this age the above rule may not apply.

In all cases of doubt about swallowed foreign bodies in children, a careful search should be made of the room. The object is sometimes found outside the child! If there is no doubt about a smooth, round, foreign body being swallowed, and the child behaves normally, then there is probably no cause for alarm. If the child behaves normally and appears well, the only need is to check that the foreign body arrives safely out of the other end, by using a 'pottie' and looking for the object. The average time is about 5–6 days. If the child appears unwell in any way, he should be taken to hospital or to a doctor. If you think that the foreign body is *inhaled* and not *swallowed*, always seek medical help by sending the casualty to hospital at once. Give nothing by mouth.

BITES

Insect bites should be treated by putting on calamine cream. A useful preventive measure is to use an insect repellent which contains diethyl toluamide, such as 'Flypel' or 'Skeeto-Stick', available from your pharmacist (chemist).

Dog bites, cat bites or other animal bites should be treated as any other dirty wound (*see* page 162). If the wound is other than trivial, it is best to have it seen by a doctor.

STINGS

If the insect leaves the sting and poison bag in the skin, remove them with your fingernail. Take care not to press on the poison bag, as pressure may squirt the poison into the wound. Then, treat as any wound by cleaning and dressing.

If there is much swelling, take the casualty to a doctor. Stings inside the mouth and on the throat can be dangerous, due to swelling which may lead to difficulty in breathing. If this happens give the casualty ice to suck and get him quickly to hospital or to a doctor.

JELLYFISH AND NETTLE STINGS

Calamine cream should be applied to the affected areas.

CRAMP

The home treatment for cramp is to contract and hold contracted as forcibly as possible the opposite set of muscles to those which are cramping, until the cramp wears off. For example, if the cramp is in the muscles of the back of the thigh (the muscles which bend the knee) the knee should be straightened as stiffly as possible, and held like this until the cramped muscles relax.

The reason why this works is because when one set of muscles contract forcibly the opposite set (in this case the cramped muscles) relax through reflex action.

'WINDING' (following a blow on the *solar plexus*)

The traditional treatment of head between the knees and pump up and down does no good. Leave the casualty in the position which he wishes to adopt (usually rolled into a ball). Reassure him that he is only winded and that in a short time he will feel better. Keep him at rest until fully recovered.

A 'STITCH' IN THE SIDE

Stop walking or running. It will pass off. No other treatment is really effective!

FRICTION BLISTERS

These may appear on the feet and hands and are often the result of some unusual activity, or may be caused by tight or ill-fitting shoes.

Cover the blister area and beyond *at once* with an adhesive plaster dressing, taking care that the dressing material is large enough to cover the blister area and a little beyond. Do not put adhesive plaster over the blister as this will only rip off the skin. If a patch is applied soon enough, further friction can be prevented and the blister may subside.

If the blister is large and uncomfortable it may be necessary to burst it. If it has burst, or if you burst it, all the dead skin must be trimmed off with scissors to the edge of the blister. Then, clean the area (*see* wounds, page 162) and apply a dressing as above, taking care not to put adhesive plaster over the blister area.

Appendix 1

RECOMMENDATIONS FOR KITS
for first-aid and for home treatment

Kit 1

First-aid kit (for first-aid = self-help and first-help)

Triangular bandage, compressed, BPC	6
No 15 BPC compressed wound-dressing – large	3
No 14 BPC compressed wound-dressing – medium	3
No 13 BPC compressed wound-dressing – small	4
Safety-pins – medium	6
Safety-pins – large	6
Paper and pencil	

This kit can be packed to fit a box sized 6 in × 3½ in × 4½ in

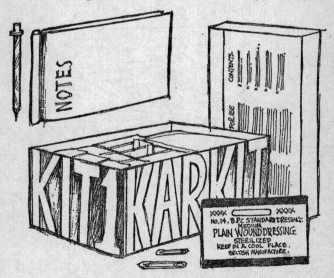

Karkit – for first-aid (self-help and first-help)

Notes

One kit should be kept at home and *another* similar kit should be kept in the car (on a boat or with your camping or caravanning gear). This kit occupies a small space, and should be duplicated and stored where it may be required. If the contents are put in a *sealed* tin, they should not deteriorate appreciably in ten years.

The contents of this kit should normally be sufficient to carry out first-aid on two casualties.

Paper and pencil are an important part of the kit. Written messages are a fairly sure method of communication and should be used to record details about the injuries found or suspected, the treatment applied, and the condition of the casualty. A note of the time at which the observations are made is also useful. It is surprising how difficult it sometimes can be to find paper and pencil; the sure thing to do is to include them as a part of the kit.

Always seal the box to keep the contents dry and to show that the kit has not been used. Replace any used articles at once.

A torch should be available with the first-aid kit.

Kit 2 – for home treatment

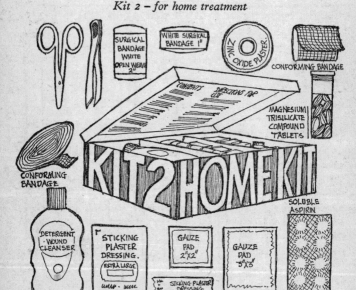

Home kit – for home treatment (only-help)

Kit 2

Home Treatment Kit	Quantity
1. 'Savlon' (ICI)	250 ml
2. Swabs, gauze 2 in × 2 in, individually wrapped, sterilized	10
Swabs, gauze 3 in × 3 in, individually wrapped, sterilized	10
Non-adherent dressing 2 in × 2 in, individually wrapped, sterile (melolin)	5
Non-adherent dressing 4 in × 4 in, individually wrapped, sterile (melolin)	5
Adhesive plaster patches with plain dressing, assorted sizes, sterile	25
3. Conforming bandage, cotton, roller, 2 in	3
Conforming bandage, cotton, roller, 3 in	3
Crêpe bandage 2 in	1
4. Soluble aspirin tablets, foil wrapped	20
Magnesium trisilicate compound tablets BPC	10
Calamine cream (Boots)	1 tube
5. Scissors 5 in, blunt pointed, stainless steel	1 pair
Tweezers (eyebrow type, spade-ended)	1 pair

Notes

1. 'Savlon' is a detergent cleaner which is suitable for cleaning all wounds, minor burns or insect bites. It should be diluted with warm water before use.

2. Dressing materials are all *sterile* and individually wrapped. Dry gauze, plain vaseline net and adhesive plaster patches (unmedicated) can be used according to suitability (*see* page 166 for details).

3. Conforming bandages are easy to apply. The crêpe bandage is for controlling bleeding inside a limb (bruising) or for ordinary bandaging.

4. (i) Soluble aspirin tablets, foil wrapped, are for the treatment of pain. The adult dose is two tablets every four hours as required. Children of seven should take one tablet every four hours. Other ages should take the amount suitable for age, counting age 14 as adult dose (2 tablets) and dividing accordingly. Aspirin

should not be given to a child under the age of two, except on the instructions of a doctor.

(ii) Magnesium trisilicate compound tablets BPC are for the relief of mild indigestion and stomach upsets. The dose is two tablets taken with a glass of milk or water.

Children under 5 should take			$\frac{1}{2}$ tablet
„	5–8	„ „	1 tablet
„	8–11	„ „	$1\frac{1}{2}$ tablets
„	over 12	„ „	2 tablets

(iii) Calamine cream is for the relief of sunburn, itchy bites, 'heat spots', or other minor skin irritation. It should be applied to the affected area(s).

5. Scissors and tweezers are essential and useful instruments. It is false economy to buy cheap plated scissors. They are never satisfactory and will soon rust or chip. Stainless scissors, given reasonable care and occasional sharpening, will last a lifetime. The scissors will be useful for cutting off dead skin, and for cutting bandages and dressings. The tweezers are essential for catching hold of and removing splinters. Both should be boiled in water for five minutes before and after use.

Container

It is a good idea to pack the kit into a container with three compartments (roughly corresponding to uses).

  (i) Wound-cleaning and dressing materials (1 and 2 in list above).
 (ii) Bandages and instruments (3 and 5 in list).
(iii) Medicines, creams, etc (4 in list).

Ample spare space should be left in part (iii) of the box. This will enable special family medicines to be included with the kit when going off on holiday. Travel-sickness preventers*, insect repellents and suntan lotions can then be carried *with* all the other home-treatment items. A box about $9\frac{1}{2}$ in × $10\frac{1}{2}$ in × $2\frac{1}{2}$ in will take these items and will leave space for extras.

If you go caravanning, sailing, or camping regularly, it is probably wise to duplicate this kit and to keep one kit at home and another in the caravan, on the boat, or with the camping gear.

* Recommended travel-sickness preventers are 'Ancolan' or 'Marzine'. Full instructions about how to take the drug are in the packet. Pregnant women should *not* take these drugs.

Appendix 2

NOTES FOR TEACHERS, AND TEACHING-AIDS

The aim should be to teach first-aid as a simple and practical subject, based on aims and principles from which the correct treatment naturally follows. Complications of all kinds should be avoided – for example, medical jargon and needless small details of anatomy, physiology and pathology. We should speak of bleeding and how to stop bleeding and not about 'the arrest of haemorrhage'. The teacher should train the class in the principles on which first-aid treatment is based in the simplest and most straightforward way possible, and give practical instruction which can easily be followed, carried out and remembered.

Much of the confusion arising in the minds of first-aiders is due to the instruction they have received. All too frequently the instruction was loaded with jargon and anatomy, appeared very complicated and was based on no system of principles or aims which they could recognize or follow. We would make a strong plea for the elimination of all irrelevant matter and for simple, straightforward teaching that can be easily understood.

A suggested outline for a course of instruction in essential first-aid is given below.

OUTLINE OF AN EIGHT-HOUR COURSE IN FIRST-AID

The aim of lectures, demonstrations and practice is to teach newcomers to be useful first-aiders. This can be achieved by four lectures, preferably from a doctor, and at least four demonstrations from a good first-aider who enjoys teaching.

PERIOD I   Introduction
(2 hours)   Chapter 1
　　　　　　Lecture:　'Priorities and the systematic approach' and 'not breathing'.
　　　　　　　　　　　Chapters 2 and 3.
　　　　　　　　　　　Demonstration and practice in mouth-to-nose and mouth-to-mouth artificial respiration, and how to feel the pulse.

PERIOD 2 *Lecture:* Bleeding and its treatment.
(2 hours)   Chapter 4.
                     Demonstration and practice in applying
                     bandages, dressings, improvisation and
                     sending for help.

PERIOD 3 *Lecture:* Unconsciousness, head injuries, burns
(2 hours)   and poisoning.
                     Chapters 5, 7, 9 and 10.
                     Demonstration of the unconscious position
                     and practice of dressings for burns.

PERIOD 4 *Lecture:* Fractures and Wet-Cold Chilling.
(2 hours)   Chapters 8 and 11.
                     Demonstration and practice in treatment of
                     fractures.

TEACHING-AIDS – FILMS

Emergency Resuscitation, Parts 1 and 2
16-mm, sound, colour.
   Part 1 deals with the reasons for doing and how to carry out
   artificial respiration by the mouth-to-nose and mouth-to-
   mouth method.
   Part 2 shows artificial respiration being carried out in emer-
   gency situations.
Made by the Royal Navy. Awarded a gold medal by the British
Medical Association. Absolutely first-class teaching film.
Available on hire or to buy from:

>   Stewart Films Ltd,
>   82 Clifton Hill,
>   London, NW8.

                                   Tel: 01–624 7296

(*Part* 3 teaches heart compression)

Don't Let Him Die
16-mm, sound, colour.
   A good presentation of basic life-saving first-aid.
   Available from:

>   Technicolour Ltd,
>   Bath Road,
>   Harmondsworth,
>   Middlesex.

TEACHING-AIDS – APPARATUS

The Ambu Manikin

for teaching artificial respiration.
Available to buy from:

>   Ambu International (UK) Ltd,
>   Brinksway Trading Estate,
>   Brinksway,
>   Stockport,
>   Cheshire.

(The Ambu Manikin may also be used to teach heart compression to advanced first-aiders.)

The Haynes Resuscitation Trainer

This is a simple and reasonably priced apparatus for teaching artificial respiration. It is well suited to the needs of schools and youth organizations.
Available to buy from:

>   Haynes Resuscitation Trainer,
>   Twyford,
>   Winchester,
>   Hampshire.

Colour transparencies

Colour transparencies of new, untreated injuries are useful for teaching. They can accustom first-aiders to the appearance of wounds, burns, fractures, dislocations and so on, and can also be used for starting a discussion about the diagnosis and correct first-aid treatment of the condition.

AUDIO-VISUAL AIDS

New Safety and First-Aid Series

Life-saving first-aid   1. *Not Breathing*   (271/1)
                            2. *Bleeding*   (271/2)
                            3. *Unconscious*   (271/3)

Each of these subjects is available both as a filmstrip (35-mm) and as an 8-mm film-loop; they show the correct first-aid for not breathing, bleeding and unconsciousness.

Safe or Sorry?   – shows injuries at work and how to pre-
                        vent them (35-mm film-strips and
                        tapes).

Injuries in the Home – shows injuries at home and how to pre-
                        vent them (35-mm film-strips and
                        tapes).

These and other colour film-strips (35-mm) and colour film-
loops (8-mm) together with other audio-visual aids for teaching
safety, accident prevention and first-aid, are available from:

>   Camera Talks Ltd,
>   31 North Row,
>   London W1

>   Tel: 01–493 2761

Poster

A poster based on the teaching in this book is available, suitable
for hanging up at home, at work, or where required. The poster
(23 in by 18 in) is entitled 'Instant First-Aid' and is printed on
stiff board in red and black. It is available from:

>   The Lyndhurst Printing Company,
>   Blackfield,
>   Southampton,
>   Hampshire.

25p plus carriage   Tel: Blackfield 2289

Leaflet on Pocket First-Aid

A pocket-sized leaflet, printed in red and black on glazed board,
called *Pocket First-Aid* is available. It covers life-saving first-aid,
first-aid to prevent worsening and first-aid for poisoning and car
crashes. The information is based on *New Essential First-Aid*
and is meant as a handy reminder.

Pocket First-Aid is also available from the Lyndhurst Printing
Company (*see* above for address).

>   25 copies   £2·50 ⎫ plus postage
>   100 copies £9·15 ⎬ and packing
>   500 copies £37·50 ⎭

Appendix 3

BOOKS FOR FURTHER READING

FIRST-AID

New Advanced First-Aid
    by A. Ward Gardner with Peter J. Roylance
      Butterworths, London
The companion volume to this, for those who wish to increase their knowledge of first-aid, both in range and depth.

Principles for First-Aid for the Injured
    by H. Proctor and P. S. London   Butterworths, London
An excellent book, the result of much experience. Not suitable for the beginner, but should be read by all who instruct in first-aid.

The Fundamentals of First-Aid   St John Ambulance,
    by Robert A. Mustard   321 Chapel Street,
                                 Ottawa, Canada.
A very good first-aid book. The 'Introductory Notes for Instructors' are a classical exposition of what first-aid is about, and what it is *not* about. We recommend it to all instructors and first-aiders.

New Safety and First-Aid
    by A. Ward Gardner and Peter J. Roylance
      Pan Books, London.
This book gives young people advice about preventing injuries as well as explaining the necessary and essential first-aid. It covers a wide field with care and thoroughness and should be on every child's and youth-leader's bookshelf.

Teaching First-Aid
    ed Stanley Miles and Peter J. Roylance
      Baillière, Tindall and Cassell, London
This volume was written by a number of experts who were asked by the Medical Commission on Accident Prevention to produce

up-to-date information on teaching first-aid. It therefore contains authoritative information and should be used by all who teach.

MEDICAL TREATMENT AT SEA OR IN REMOTE PLACES

The Ship Captain's Medical Guide	HMSO, London
The Ship's Medicine Chest and First-Aid at Sea	US Government Printing Office, Washington
International Guide for Ships	WHO, Geneva

All of these books are designed to give instruction in what to do when a doctor is not available. They assume that medical supplies such as are – and have to be – carried by the ship are available. The choice of book would depend largely on individual preference and nationality! Perhaps all would be useful.

Exploration Medicine edited by O. G. Edholm and A. L. Bacharach	John Wright & Sons Ltd, Bristol

This book surveys the medical problems which arise in planning and carrying out expeditions. It includes much useful information on supplies, equipment, camp hygiene, and disease prevention and treatment. The book is a must for modern explorers.

A Traveller's Guide to Health by J. M. Adam	Hodder & Stoughton, London

A foreword states that this is 'a practical, down-to-earth, simple book which could be used by those without medical knowledge who were out of range of medical help'. The book covers the same sort of ground as *Exploration Medicine* and is a companion volume covering the same subjects, but written for the non-expert. The book is small and easily portable and can be recommended with confidence to all who travel to remote places and need a medical guide.

HOW THE BODY IS CONSTRUCTED AND HOW IT FUNCTIONS
(Anatomy and Physiology)

The Human Body by C. Bibby and I. T. Morison	Penguin, London

Written for children, but suitable for adults. A very clear exposi-

tion in short compass of the basic facts about the human body.
Very well illustrated.

Basic Anatomy and Physiology   John Murray, London
   by R. G. Q. Rowett
This text is basic in the sense that it is not for doctors. It should,
however, be more than adequate for anybody who wishes to
learn anatomy for non-specialist purposes. The anatomy part of
the book is well done and the illustrations are good. Physiology
is rather glossed over by comparison and is less well presented.

Anatomy, Physiology and Hygiene
   by J. K. Raeburn, H. A. Raeburn
   and H. M. Gration   John Murray, London
A useful book for anyone who wishes to understand the basics of
human biology. Written mainly with nurses in mind, but also
suitable for any course in human biology up to GCE level. The
illustrations are adequate and the balance between anatomy and
physiology is well maintained.

Index

HEALTH AND FAMILY AFFAIRS

COOKERY AND HOME MANAGEMENT

Robert Carrier. All colour illustrated. ($5'' \times 5\frac{3}{8}''$)
DINNER PARTY MENUS   20p

LUNCHEON PARTY MENUS   20p

BREAKFAST AND BRUNCH PARTY MENUS   20p

BARBECUE PARTY MENUS   20p

CHILDREN'S PARTY MENUS   20p

SUPPER PARTY MENUS   20p

Mrs Beeton
ALL ABOUT COOKERY (illus.)   37½p

Claire Loewenfeld & Philip a Back
HERBS FOR HEALTH AND COOKERY   35p

John Doxat
**BOOTH'S HANDBOOK OF COCKTAILS AND
MIXED DRINKS**   25p

Miss Read
MISS READ'S COUNTRY COOKING   30p

SPORTS AND PASTIMES

CLASSICS SELECTION

A series of the most popular books by the world's greatest authors. Each volume is completely unabridged and contains an analytic introduction and notes, often by a famous author.

Jane Austen
NORTHANGER ABBEY   25p

PERSUASION   25p

PRIDE AND PREJUDICE   25p

EMMA   30p

Arnold Bennett
THE OLD WIVES' TALE   37½p

Charlotte Bronte
JANE EYRE   25p

Emily Bronte
WUTHERING HEIGHTS   25p

Wilkie Collins
THE MOONSTONE   30p

These and other PAN Books are obtainable from all book-sellers and newsagents. If you have any difficulty please send purchase price plus 5p postage to P.O. Box 11, Falmouth, Cornwall.
While every effort is made to keep prices low, it is sometimes necessary to increase prices at short notice. PAN Books reserve the right to show new retail prices on covers which may differ from those advertised in the text or elsewhere.